Plastic Surgery
for Trauma

Plastic Surgery for Trauma

The Essential Survival Guide

Edited by

Dorian Hobday, MA, MBBS, MRCS
Specialist Registrar, Department of Plastic and Reconstructive Surgery, Barts and the Royal London Hospital, UK

Ted Welman, MBBS, MRCS
Specialist Registrar, Department of Plastic and Reconstructive Surgery, Barts and the Royal London Hospital, UK

Maxim D. Horwitz, MBChB FRCS (Orth) DipHandSurg
Consultant Hand Surgeon, Chelsea and Westminster Hospital, UK. Honorary Clinical Senior Lecturer, Imperial College London, UK

Gurjinderpal Singh Pahal, MBChB (Ed), FRCS (Plast)
Consultant Plastic and Reconstructive Surgeon, Clinical Lead, Barts and the Royal London Hospital, UK

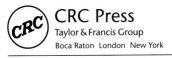

CRC Press
Taylor & Francis Group
Boca Raton London New York

CRC Press is an imprint of the
Taylor & Francis Group, an **informa** business

First edition published 2022
by CRC Press
6000 Broken Sound Parkway NW, Suite 300, Boca Raton, FL 33487-2742

and by CRC Press
2 Park Square, Milton Park, Abingdon, Oxon, OX14 4RN

CRC Press is an imprint of Taylor & Francis Group, LLC

ISBN: 9780367757366 (hbk)
ISBN: 9780367750701 (pbk)
ISBN: 9781003163770 (ebk)

DOI: 10.1201/9781003163770

Typeset in Minion Pro
by KnowledgeWorks Global Ltd.

Contents

v

Chapter 9 ■ Burns   139

Chapter 10 ■ Facial Trauma   165

Chapter 11 ■ Free Flaps   179

Chapter 12 ■ Career Development   187

REFERENCES, 197

INDEX, 201

Preface

This book covers the immediate assessment and management of common plastic and reconstructive surgery emergencies and referrals. It is conceived as a concise guide rather than a comprehensive textbook, in order to be easily utilised by those new to the speciality. As such, the emphasis is on immediate management and the steps required to prepare a patient for definitive management.

Written by junior plastic surgeons who can recall what it is like to start in plastics, its intention is to prepare and support house officers in their challenging first weeks and months of working in plastic surgery, and to give them the insights that would normally only be acquired from being 'on the job'.

We hope you enjoy your journey in plastic surgery.

DH and TW

Acknowledgements

To GSP who has moulded our lives and careers with his dedication to us.

Thanks to our partners, Miranda and Eric, without whose support this book would not have become a reality.

Thanks to the Royal London Plastics family who assisted in gathering cases for the book: Harry Burton, Sajeda Ismail, Rebecca Harsten, Isabelle Citron, Omar Abbassi, Jason Roberts, Josh Michaels, Roxanna Lord, Isabelle Drummond, Tonderai Mutsago, Jim O'Hagan and Harriet Middleton. Special thanks to Dardan Popova for his input on the photography and to Kamal El-Ali for his input on the drawings.

Thanks to the team at Taylor & Francis for their guidance and support.

TW, DH

I also dedicate this to my late mother, whose support of my wandering path was absolute.

DH

Contributors

Chapter 8

Dardan Popova
The Royal London Hospital
Barts Health NHS Trust
United Kingdom

William Thompson
The Royal London Hospital
Barts Health NHS Trust
United Kingdom

Ahmed Mahmoud ElBaz
The Royal London Hospital
Barts Health NHS Trust
United Kingdom

Chapter 9

Gary Masterton
The Countess of Chester
    Hospital NHS Trust
United Kingdom

Cyrus Talwar
Plastic Surgery Registrar
Chelsea & Westminster
    Hospital
United Kingdom

Harriet Middleton
Plastic Surgery and Burns
    Clinical Nurse Specialist
The Royal London Hospital
United Kingdom

Chapter 10

Zak Vinnicombe
Department of Plastic and
    Reconstructive Surgery
St. George's Hospital
London, United Kingdom

Chapter 11

Amir Mahmoud Mohamed Labib Ghareib
Plastic Surgery Registrar
St. George's University
    Hospital NHS Trust
United Kingdom

Kerri Cooper
Imperial College
    NHS Trust
United Kingdom

Chapters 1–7 & Chapter 12

Dorian Hobday
Specialist Registrar
Barts and the Royal
London Hospital
United Kingdom

Ted Welman
Specialist Registrar Barts
and the Royal London
Hospital United Kingdom

On Training

Gurjinderpal Singh Pahal

As plastic surgeons, we are privileged to be trained in the painstaking art of reconstruction. Restoration of form, function and aesthetics is paramount, and reintegration into family, society and the workplace are equally as important. From Sushruta to Tagliacozzi, and in more recent times, from Gillies to McIndoe, reconstructive surgery has always found its roots in solving problems, especially those caused by trauma, infection or cancer. The aforementioned principles underpin the ethos of our specialty and, with the evolution of surgical practice and enhancement of technology, plastic surgeons of the modern era are able to achieve results that would have been inconceivable to their predecessors.

Reconstructive surgery requires the perceptive eye of an artist coupled with the delicate hand of a craftsman – it is surgery at its most refined. Principles such as planning in reverse, appreciation of geometrical shapes and anatomical sub-units, restoring like-with-like and the philosophy of 'manoeuvring the Apostles', or borrowing from Peter to pay Paul, make this specialty an innovative art form. Knowledge of anatomy is key and forms the foundation of not only plastic and reconstructive surgery but also surgery in general. Understanding the layers and blood supply of skin and its underlying structures, appreciation of bloodless tissue planes and having knowledge of scars and where best to place them, from both a functional and cosmetic perspective, should be knowledge that is inherent to any plastic surgeon.

As I have progressed through the ranks within plastic surgery, firstly as a trainee and now as a consultant trainer and mentor, I have come to an understanding that the training process is much more than the act of surgery itself. The key elements of work ethic, operating principles, and unit geography and demographics play important roles in enabling training to take place. In this introduction I will touch on these elements in turn.

WORK ETHIC

The personality and work ethic of a trainee has a huge impact on learning, and excellence in training is achieved through a mutually respectful mentor-mentee relationship. Keeping abreast of knowledge, having the desire to learn new techniques and consistently improving one's surgical skill and dexterity make training fun, enjoyable and rewarding. Surgical decorum such as punctuality, adequate preparation for upcoming operative lists and engagement in planning of cases should not be underestimated in terms of creating the ideal atmosphere for training to take place. This 'surgical etiquette' is equally as important as the physical act of surgery itself.

It is wise to treat everybody involved with patient care and surgical training with respect and courtesy, and this includes both nursing and surgical teams, as well as contemporaries in ancillary specialties. This relationship works both ways; if you exhibit respect and dedication to your training, your mentors will recognise this and you will be rewarded by their unfaltering support and dedication to you as their trainees. I pass on the following aide-mémoir to my juniors that I was taught by my former mentors during my own training: Always be **affable, able** and **available**.

Being **affable** to those around you goes a long way in the hospital environment. This applies not just to your behaviour with fellow surgeons and patients, but to every hospital professional you interact with. Being a positive presence engenders positive behaviour in return.

The aforementioned qualities of being prepared and organised go some way towards being **able**, but it is also vital for a trainee to reflect on their performance as a surgeon on a daily basis and work out how to improve. If you are actively addressing your weak points, your trainers will remain engaged. If you are not, and make the same mistake repeatedly, they may lose interest.

Being **available** is about being responsive and willing to help. If you promptly respond to calls or messages, your colleagues will know that they can rely on you when they need help or advice. If you are someone who is willing to 'pitch in' when the system is stretched, or to go above and beyond to assist with a difficult case, then again colleagues will know that they can rely on you, and this will build their trust and respect for you.

OPERATING PRINCIPLES

The Royal London Upper Limb Trauma Fellowship was introduced some years ago to formalise the transition from junior fellow to numbered registrar with a National Training Number (NTN). To date, all fellows that have successfully completed this apprenticeship have secured an NTN and have been ranked in the top 5 Nationally. This is through their own sheer dedication, commitment and desire to learn and improve, coupled with an unparalleled exposure to a high volume of hand trauma of varying complexity, and one-on-one consultant supervision for each and every case. The realistic expectation is that the fellow operates on between 20 and 24 patients a week divided between parallel lists of fractures and soft tissues. Though the traditional nature of the surgical firm has become less common, this training relationship can be built if a trainee and a consultant have the will to do so, and I would encourage you to seek this out wherever you can. What follows is a summary of what I pass on to my trainees.

An operation is more likely to succeed if operating theatre ergonomics are optimised. Even the simplest of tasks such as adequate positioning of the operative light, the set-up of the x-ray machine and the scrub trolley, the application of surgical drapes in a neat and ordered fashion and the height of the bed and surgical stool allow the surgeon to be comfortable and harbours efficiency. Looking and feeling the part not only builds the confidence of the surgeon, but also that of the theatre staff in that surgeon. An ideal operating room environment allows one to focus on operating without distraction, which maximises the chances of performing the operation well. Conversely, if the surgeon feels awkward in theatre – hunched, struggling to visualise the operating field, with equipment not in easy reach – they are setting up themselves and the rest of the team to fail.

When operating, or when thinking about any given operation, I break down the steps into smaller manageable components and perform a mental 'dress-rehearsal' of that operation. This enables the surgeon to adequately perfect each step individually, and with experience and repetition, those steps seamlessly flow into a crescendo of an operation completed from skin to skin. An example of an elementary surgical roadmap could include steps such as planning of the surgical approach and incision, dissection technique, operative repair, haemostasis, closure, local anaesthesia and dressings. Of course, each of these broad steps can be expanded into multiple smaller elements, and it is the mastery of all of these elements that equates to surgical competency. Moreover, I don't use a large number of instruments to operate with, and find it better to have a small armamentarium of instruments that one is confident and competent with. I also find using the scalpel as a tool to incise as well as dissect creates confidence, speed and an extremely neat operating field.

Optimal performance of a procedure requires an understanding of the delicacy required at each step. I explain this to trainees as the principle of '**crawl, walk, run**'. There is no point in crawling when you should run, e.g. closure of skin, and equally it is foolhardy to run when you should crawl, e.g. dissection of a perforator during free tissue transfer. Be aware that one begets the other; in the open fixation of a metacarpal fracture, e.g. a rapid, confident and meticulous dissection down to the fracture site while respecting vital layers such as the periosteum *creates the time that is needed* for the key step of reduction and fixation of the fracture.

The old adage of **'see, do, teach'** still stands; however, the number that is seen, done and taught at each separate stage depends entirely on the complexity of the procedure, as well as the surgical exposure and knowledge of the trainee. I structure my apprenticeship so that the apprentice assists me and learns the principles of operating for 3 months. The roles are then reversed, and for the next 3 months I assist my trainee as they start to put what they have observed into practice. This period of 'consultant as assistant' is crucial as it allows me to supervise their progress, and to reinforce their learning as they begin to 'teach' me out loud what they have learned. For the remaining 6 months, the trainees have built up the confidence and experience to run the lists independently, teaching the juniors who assist them, while having the safety net of the un-scrubbed consultant sitting in theatre.

Finally, learning is crucially supported by following up patients in the outpatient environment to close the loop of the patient journey, including dressing clinics and therapy appointments. It is mandatory for my fellow to plan and attend the hand trauma 1-week post-operative clinic, along with myself and the hand therapy team, to see our outcomes. They see the good, the bad *and* the ugly results, and learning is built through discussion and appraisal of such cases. If a surgeon does not follow up their patients, they truly have no way of knowing if the intervention they have made has been a success or a failure. It also gives one the opportunity to provide patients with continuity of care that defines best surgical practice.

GEOGRAPHY AND DEMOGRAPHICS

Each plastic surgical unit has its own unique identity which stems from the geography of where it is located and the demographics of the population it serves. The types and acuity of cases that present to the department, the overall caseload and the variety of pathology that the department manages, feed into the atmosphere and ethos of that department.

For example, at The Royal London Hospital in East London, we manage a complex cohort of patients from a wide variety of ethnic and social backgrounds. Levels of knife and gun crime in the surrounding area are among the highest in the United Kingdom if not in Europe, and as a result there is a high caseload of upper limb injuries and peripheral nerve injuries related to sharp trauma. As a Major Trauma Centre (MTC), we also manage lower limb reconstruction as well as complex traumatic wounds elsewhere on the body, and microsurgical reconstruction has become the bread and butter of our department for the management of major trauma. Working alongside other specialties, such as general surgery, orthopaedics, gynae-oncology, paediatrics and cardiothoracics, we also carry out a high volume of combined reconstructive cases ranging from the most straightforward interventions to the most highly complex and innovative reconstructions. Being aware of these factors is important as not only do different units offer different training opportunities, but different units suit different individuals to a greater or lesser extent.

Finding out in advance what a unit offers, and the nature of the working atmosphere, may allow one to seek institutions that match one's learning needs and personality.

Finally, never forget that with surgical training comes a huge responsibility to your patients. Respect them, be kind to them, listen to them, care for them as you would a family member and do your utmost for them and their families. Be skilful, have humility and never stop learning. Operating on patients is a privilege, and should always be treated as such.

CHAPTER 1

Hand Assessment

In acute hand trauma and hand infection, the combination of the three elements of history, examination and imaging (if required) will inform your management plan.

Do not forget to check for other injuries or medical issues as these may influence management. Around 7% of poly-trauma patients have injuries to the upper limb [a], so bear in mind that your patient may require treatment for these other potentially more urgent injuries prior to the definitive management of the hand injury. Equally, a severe infection to the upper limb may be linked to other significant medical issues, so you may need to ensure your patient is admitted under the care of the medical team as well as plastics.

HISTORY

It is important to find out the *timing* of injuries as this can influence the urgency of operative management, both in bony and soft tissue injuries. You will need to take a

DOI: 10.1201/9781003163770-1

1

focussed medical and social history (Table 1.1) as this may influence the management plan.

EXAMINATION

Following the steps of *Inspection, Palpation* and *Functional assessment* (Look, Feel, Move) guards against missing steps of the examination. Equally, even if an issue

TABLE 1.1 Hand History

Question	Comments
Mechanism of injury	**Lacerations: Was it a slicing or stabbing mechanism?** Stabs are more likely to damage deep structures and may leave a deceptively small wound.
	What was the object that caused the injury? Glass or metal fragments can be seen on X-ray, whereas wood is less visible. Dirty objects have a higher chance of causing wound contamination requiring formal washout.
	What was position of the hand at time of injury? Clues to structures likely damaged, and that there may be a mismatch of laceration site to underlying structures damaged, especially in tendon injuries.
	Crush injuries: What was the object and speed? Severe crush can devitalise tissue and also cause compartment syndrome.
Time of injury	**Delay to presentation may affect your management.** An animal bite from 2 days prior will likely be infected and require formal washout, admission and IV antibiotics, whereas it may be sufficient to washout a same-day bite and discharge on oral antibiotics.

(Continued)

TABLE 1.1 Hand History *(Continued)*

Question	Comments
	A delay in the presentation of tendon/nerve injury may require you to expedite their operative management. Operative repairs in older fractures are more challenging due to callous formation as the bone heals. **If there has been a delay, then why is this?** There may be confounding factors that prevented immediate presentation. In paediatrics, never forget to consider non-accidental injury.
Initial management completed	**Have tetanus/antibiotics already been given? Has imaging been performed? Has the wound been appropriately washed?**
Medical history to include	**Previous hand injuries? Diabetic?**
Drug history + allergies	Anti-coagulants may affect surgical planning.
Social history to include	**Smoking status?** This – along with diabetic status – has significant effect on wound healing. **Tetanus and COVID vaccination status? Socioeconomic situation?** Need to return to work/inability to engage with hand therapy may influence management.
Hand history	**Hand dominance? Line of work?** Self-employed manual labourers may opt for the fastest return to work solution over other options, e.g. terminalisation of an amputated digit vs. replantation. **Hobbies involving hands?**
Psych/safeguarding issues	**Consider if patient needs to be seen by psych,** e.g. deliberate self-harm, or the safeguarding team-abuse.
If potential emergency surgery	**Time patient last ate and drank.**

appears localised to the hand, do not forget to expose the arm to the elbow for completeness. Always examine both hands – what appears to be abnormal in an injured hand (rotation or swelling) may reveal itself to be normal when compared to the other hand. Be clear in your findings as, once the dressing is back on, you will be required to document them accurately from memory. Photographs (if taken using GDPR and appropriate governance) can assist with this and facilitate onward handover or management discussions without further dressing changes.

In lacerations where there is uncertainty if tendons or nerves have been damaged, it is often worth taking the time to anaesthetise the area of injury with a local block to allow thorough examination with a reasonably clean field. This not only improves your assessment of damaged structures but also keeps the patient comfortable and will permit you to perform a thorough washout in the emergency department. This should be done AFTER assessing sensation.

Inspection

Site and type of injury (crush/degloving/nailbed, etc.)

- Skin
  - Discolouration (erythema, white, blue)
  - Lacerations/wounds
    - Actively bleeding?
    - Clean/contaminated?
    - Skin loss/degloving?

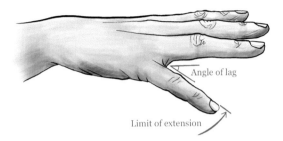

FIGURE 1.1   Extensor lag of little finger due to 5th metacarpal fracture.

- Swelling or deformity
  - Asymmetry
  - Angulation, rotation
  - Posturing of the hand (e.g. Figures 1.1 and 1.2)
  - Previous injury

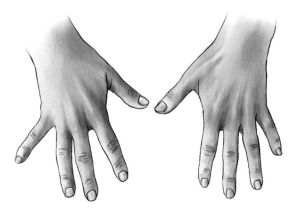

FIGURE 1.2   Asymmetry of little finger suggestive of P1 fracture.

Palpation

- Temperature
  - Warm – infection/inflammation
  - Cool – arterial insufficiency (check capillary refill time and pulses)
- Tenderness
- Surface irregularities (? foreign bodies)
- Swelling (oedema, joint effusion)
- Ligament stability (if concern of ligament disruption: Is there an endpoint?) (Figure 1.3a,b)
- Sensory assessment (if numbness, how numb exactly? Establish baseline of normal feeling "10/10" outside the zone of injury then ask the patient to compare to the area of reduced sensation (Figures 1.4 and 1.5)
- Moisture (nerve damage may inhibit ability to sweat. Nerve damage also inhibits the ability for wrinkle formation when immersed in water for a few minutes. This can be a useful test in children unable to comment on numbness.)
- Crepitus (fractures), clicking or snapping (tendonitis)

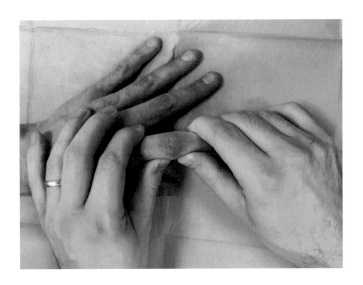

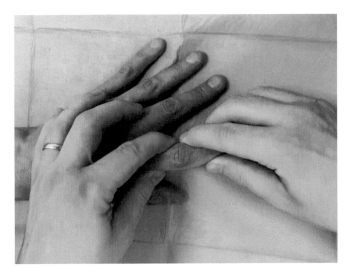

FIGURE 1.3 (a) Testing ulnar collateral ligaments of PIPJ. (b) Testing radial collateral ligaments of PIPJ.

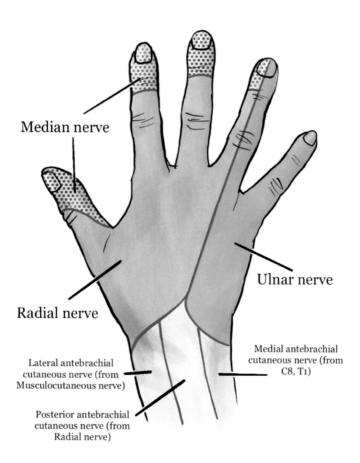

FIGURE 1.4 Dorsal dermatomes of the hand.

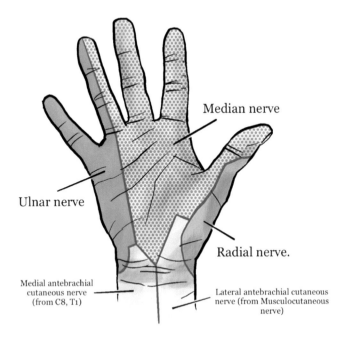

Median nerve

Ulnar nerve

Radial nerve.

Medial antebrachial
cutaneous nerve
(from C8, T1)

Lateral antebrachial cutaneous
nerve (from Musculocutaneous
nerve)

FIGURE 1.5   Volar dermatomes of the hand.

Functional Assessment

- Test active and passive range of motion of the fingers, thumb and wrist to test specific tendons or specific nerves (Table 1.2). Document if any movements are weak or painful as this may indicate *partial* tendon or nerve injury.

- A good rapid tendon assessment which shows a complete division of a flexor or an extensor can

TABLE 1.2   Motor Assessment of Hand

Nerve	Function
Median nerve	
• Intrinsic	Thumb palmar abduction (Figure 1.7)
• Extrinsic	Flexor pollicis longus
	All flexor digitorum superficialis (FDS) (Figure 1.8)
	Flexor digitorum profundus (FDP) to index (Figure 1.9)
	Flexor carpi radialis
Ulnar nerve	
• Intrinsic	Abduction/adduction of fingers (Figure 1.10)
• Extrinsic	Hypothenar muscles
	FDP to little
	Flexor carpi ulnaris
Radial nerve	
• Extrinsic	Wrist extension
	Finger extension
	Thumb extension (Figure 1.11)

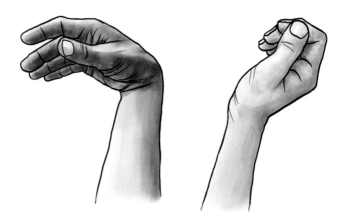

FIGURE 1.6   Tenodesis or natural cascade of fingers.

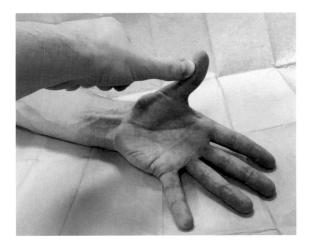

FIGURE 1.7   Testing thumb abduction – Patient abducts against resistance. Tests median intrinsic function. Contraction of the muscle bulk of the thenar eminence should be palpable.

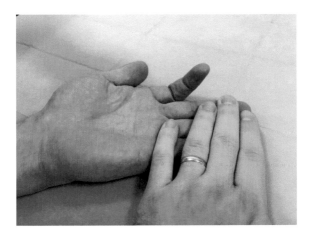

FIGURE 1.8   Testing FDS tendon – Isolate the finger by holding down the others and ask patient to flex.

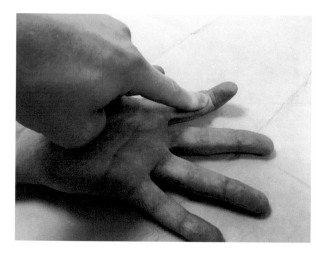

FIGURE 1.9   Testing FDP tendon – Hold down the finger over P2 and ask the patient to flex the end of their finger.

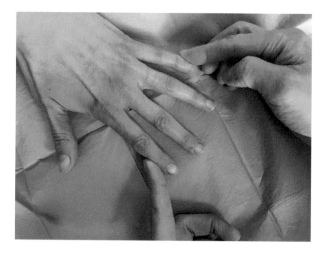

FIGURE 1.10   Testing finger abduction – Patient abducts against resistance. Tests ulnar intrinsic function.

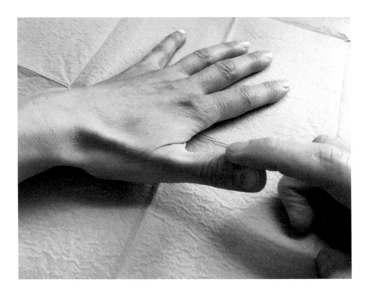

FIGURE 1.11   Testing EPL tendon – Ask patient to rest palm flat on the table and lift thumb towards the ceiling.

be achieved by checking tenodesis (Figure 1.6) – passively flex and extend the wrist and observe the cascade of the hand while the patient is relaxed (compare with other hand if any uncertainty). If the cascade is normal in flexion and extension, it is unlikely that there is complete division of extrinsic tendon(s).

- Test individual tendons as appropriate.

- A seemingly minimally displaced (on X-ray) metacarpal or phalangeal fracture may result in a significantly rotated digit. This can result in scissoring – overlapping of one finger on another upon flexion of the fingers into the fist position (Figure 1.12).

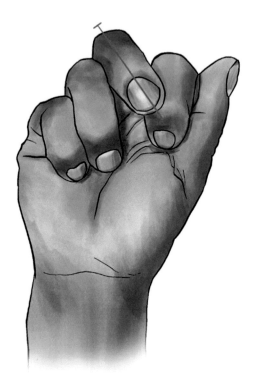

FIGURE 1.12   Scissoring of middle finger due to fracture.

- Test for scissoring of the affected digit by actively (or if this is difficult passively) flexing the digit to see if the movement reveals significant scissoring. Compare it to the normal side to be sure.

COVID

The onset of COVID has led to changes in the management of hand injuries designed to minimise patient contact and to allow surgery to continue with reduced anaesthetic coverage. These changes have been implemented to varying degrees across different units so, as previously mentioned, check the specifics when you join your unit. In hand surgery there has been an increase in the use of wide awake local anaesthetic no tourniquet (WALANT) surgery, which can be performed without an anaesthetist and which involves using larger volumes of local anaesthetic + adrenaline to achieve an anaesthetised, blood-free operating field.

It is good to be aware of the overarching BSSH (British Society for Surgery of the Hand) COVID recommendations which are as follows:

- Reconfigure into a one-stop shop including hand therapy.

- Use WALANT or regional block for all suitable procedures.

- Use absorbable sutures.

- Facilitate hand therapy instructions at first visit and minimise further face-to-face contact.

- Set up video consultations for surgical and hand therapy follow-up.

- Ensure there is a safe system of pre-operative swabbing and self-isolation as per the NICE guidelines.

CHAPTER 2

Local Anaesthetic Blocks

Local anaesthetic (LA) has many applications both in and out of the operating theatre. In the on-call context it is useful for facilitating pain-free wound examination, drainage of infection and for minor operations, such as wound closure and nailbed repairs (Table 2.1).

Before giving LA, it is essential to check the allergy status of the patient. It is worth warning the patient that the anaesthetic itself will cause some pain and a feeling of pressure as it is administered. Also explain that once the anaesthetic has taken effect it will eliminate sharp pain but that they will still be able to sense movement and touch.

Maximal analgesic effect takes approximately 15 minutes for all local anaesthetics. The vasoconstrictive action of adrenaline takes longer (25–30 minutes). It is therefore advisable to wait after giving the anaesthetic

DOI: 10.1201/9781003163770-2

TABLE 2.1   Local Anaesthetic Characteristics [b] [c]

Anaesthetic Agent	Maximum Dose, mg/kg	Onset of Action	Duration of Action
Lidocaine	3	<2 min	30–60 min
Lidocaine with adrenaline	6	<2 min	60–90 min
Bupivacaine	2	5–10 min	240–480 min
Bupivacaine with adrenaline	2	5–10 min	360–720 min
Prilocaine	6	5 min	30–90 min
Prilocaine with adrenaline	8	5 min	60–120 min

before starting any procedure. In practice we advise: Administer the LA before going to gather the things you need – dressings, suture pack, etc. Note that using a LA mixed with adrenaline not only prolongs the anaesthesia time but also reduces bleeding at the wound site due to the vasoconstrictive properties of adrenaline.

Mixing short- and long-acting anaesthetics (e.g. lidocaine and bupivacaine) gives the advantages of both, i.e. rapid onset and a longer half-life. The addition of 10% by volume of 8.4% sodium bicarbonate solution neutralises the acidity of the local anaesthetic and has been demonstrated to make the administration less painful. In practical terms this means adding 1 mL of 8.4% sodium bicarbonate to 10 mL of local anaesthetic to total 11 mL. Warming the anaesthetic to room temperature, using a small gauge needle, and injecting slowly have also been shown to increase patient comfort [d].

Caution must be taken to avoid intravenous injection of LA by *always withdrawing the plunger prior to injecting* in order to ensure the needle tip is not in a vessel. This process must be repeated every time you reposition the needle. If the patient experiences a very sharp pain, the needle tip may be in a nerve and it should therefore be slightly withdrawn before proceeding.

DIGITAL BLOCK/RING BLOCK

Historically, it has been common practice to avoid the inclusion of adrenaline when administering a digital block due to the concern of digital ischaemia. This has been discredited and is now a well-established technique in most areas of hand surgery so don't be afraid to use adrenaline containing LA solutions (e.g. Xylocaine: pre-mixed 1% lidocaine + 1:200,000 adrenaline) [e].

In the on-call context, digital LA blocks permit the examination of wounds and repair of nailbed injuries or simple lacerations. In theatres they can be used for the repair of extensor tendons and procedures such as digit terminalisation or fixation of distal phalanx fractures.

Eight millilitres of LA is normally sufficient to block a digit in an average adult. In a small or paediatric hand less is required. Inject with a fine gauge needle (Orange 25G or Blue 22G). Gently pinch the skin over the knuckle then inject 4–6 mL subcutaneously (Figure 2.1). You will see this fill the space at the dorsal base of the finger from where it will diffuse around the finger. Following this, ask the patient to turn over their hand so you can inject a further 2–4 mL on the volar aspect just proximal to the crease at the base of finger (Figure 2.2). Do this injection with the needle at a right angle to the skin. Note: The volar injection is more painful so warn the patient (Figure 2.3).

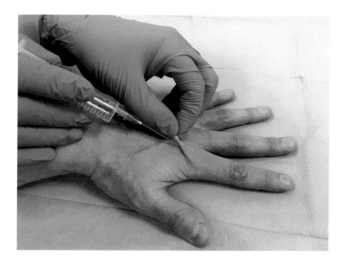

FIGURE 2.1   Dorsal element of digital block.

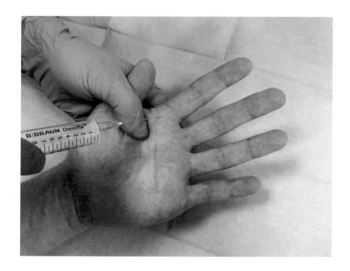

FIGURE 2.2   Volar element of digital block.

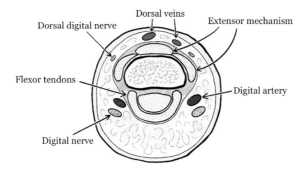

FIGURE 2.3   Cross-sectional anatomy of proximal finger. Note: Majority of sensation is via larger volar digital nerves.

Note: There are multiple ways to administer a ring block so depending on your experience and your seniors input, you will develop a preferred technique.

WRIST BLOCKS

Wrist blocks allow individual blocking of the median, ulnar and radial nerves at the level of the wrist to anaesthetise whole nerve territories. When administering wrist blocks, be aware that there is crossover between dermatomes, so it is prudent to block more than one nerve even if you think your area of injury is specific to one nerve territory. Use a needle that is long enough to reach the target nerve (blue 22 gauge is well suited). As large vessels lie close to the ulnar and radial nerves it is particularly important to remember to withdraw the plunger before injecting to ensure the needle is not in a vessel. Do not be deterred by this – wrist blocks are generally safe and effective if this simple step is followed. Be aware the time for the anaesthetic to take full effect is longer than in a digital block.

Median Nerve Block

Identify the palmaris longus and flexor carpi radialis tendons just proximal to the wrist crease by asking the patient to flex their wrist. Then with the wrist relaxed insert the needle between them at 90 degrees to the skin (Figure 2.4). You may feel a 'pop' as you pass through the flexor retinaculum into the carpal tunnel. If the patient reports sharp pain or tingling in the median nerve distribution, it likely indicates the tip of the needle is in the nerve so withdraw a little prior to injecting. Inject the LA within the carpal tunnel. As you withdraw, it can help to raise a superficial bleb of anaesthetic distally to block the palmar cutaneous branch of the median nerve. Between 5 and 10 mL is sufficient for the block.

Radial Nerve Block

At the level of the wrist, it is the superficial branch of the radial nerve that requires blocking so it is a subcutaneous

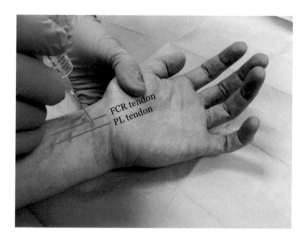

FIGURE 2.4   Median nerve block.

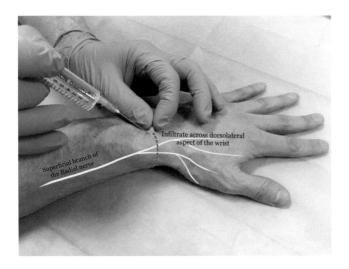

Infiltrate across dorsolateral
aspect of the wrist

Superficial branch of
the Radial nerve

FIGURE 2.5   Radial nerve block.

injection. Introduce the needle just proximal to the anatomical snuffbox and advance it at the subcutaneous level
to the dorsal midpoint of the wrist, injecting 5–7 mL of LA
as you go (Figure 2.5). This block should raise a confluent
subcutaneous bleb to confirm you are at the right depth.

Ulnar Nerve Block

Identify the flexor carpi ulnaris tendon proximal to the
wrist crease and insert your needle under this tendon in a
volar and radial direction (Figure 2.6). To achieve this, you
may require the patient to slightly lift and hyper pronate
their hand. The nerve lies deep and radial to flexor carpi
ulnaris with the ulnar artery radial to the nerve (Figure 2.7).
Having ensured the needle tip is not in the ulnar artery,
inject 5–7 mL of anaesthetic as you withdraw.

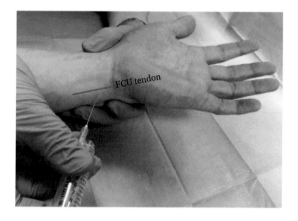

FIGURE 2.6   Ulnar nerve block.

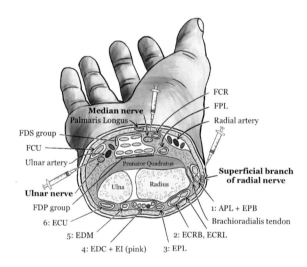

FIGURE 2.7   Anatomy of wrist proximal to the carpal tunnel + injection sites for wrist block. Note location of nerves in relation to tendons and arteries.

CHAPTER 3

Hand Infections

Infections of the hand are common and account for a high proportion of hand presentations seen in the emergency department (ED). Prompt diagnosis and management are key to achieving optimal outcomes and limiting long-term stiffness/loss of function. Missed or poorly managed serious infections can result in amputation.

Hand infections most commonly occur post-traumatic injury, though the trauma may be minor such as an insect bite or a scratch. A full medical history is important as a number of patient groups are particularly susceptible to infection and tend to have worse outcomes (Table 3.1). This cohort requires more aggressive treatment and closer monitoring [f].

Staphylococcus aureus and *Streptococcus* are the most frequent causative pathogens. Microbiology cultures are important in targeting therapy so ensure a pus sample is taken before antibiotics are commenced. Increased-risk

DOI: 10.1201/9781003163770-3

TABLE 3.1   Medical Conditions with Increased Risk in Hand Infections

---

Diabetes mellitus

- Higher rates of deep space infection, amputations and necrotising fasciitis
- Hyperglycaemia favours bacterial proliferation
- Peripheral neuropathy may mask pain and thus delay presentation
- Diabetes with renal failure is especially morbid with high amputation rates for extremity infection [g]

Immunosuppressed

- Transplant patients
- AIDS
- Autoimmune disorders

Alcohol and drug abuse

Renal failure

Malnutrition

---

patients or patients who present with chronic infection are more likely to have gram negative or unusual infective organisms so in this cohort consider sending tissue for fungal cultures also.

In your history ask about systemic symptoms such as fevers or rigors. Ask also about pain or swelling in the axilla as this may suggest that the infection has spread. On examination of any hand infection ensure the arm is fully exposed to avoid missing the presence of lymphangitis or the proximal spread of cellulitis. If cellulitis is present, mark and date its outer boundary so progression can be monitored. If there is any suspicion of systemic involvement, blood tests should be sent to assess severity of infection and to serve as a baseline. X-rays of the affected limb may be required to rule out the presence of a foreign body or, in the case of a deep seated or chronic infection, to investigate the possibility of osteomyelitis.

Fluctuant swellings with purulent discharge will require drainage and washout with saline either in ED or (depending on severity of infection and the patient) in theatres. Local anaesthetic can be helpful in facilitating the drainage but is best given AWAY from the site of infection to avoid spreading the infection. Recent studies have demonstrated that tap water can be as effective as saline for washout [h]. If there is a significant collection it is practical to do the initial drainage and washout under running water in a sink before completing saline washing, assessment and dressing of the wound in the normal way. If the infection is loculated, it is very important to break the loculations to release all pockets of infection. The site of infection should NOT be closed as this generally leads to recurrence of the collection.

Infections with a sizable collection or significant cellulitis will require admission for intravenous antibiotics and monitoring. Superficial or localised infections with mild cellulitis can often be managed in the community with oral antibiotics.

Following your assessment, drainage and washout, ensure the following management steps are completed in all hand infections:

- Dressing and splinting of the affected hand in the position of safe immobility (POSI – Figure 3.1)– unless involving finger only

- Strict elevation of the limb

  - Inpatient: Bradford sling

  - Outpatient: Polysling/high arm sling

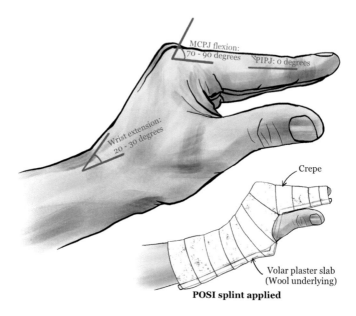

FIGURE 3.1   Position of safe immobilisation (POSI). Immobilise as above with a volar plaster slab from the mid forearm to the fingertip. This position serves to minimise the contracture of joint ligaments and the intrinsic muscles of the hand.

- Prophylactic tetanus (if patient not covered) for all penetrating wounds

- Immediate commencement of broad-spectrum antibiotics as per trust guidelines (intravenous or oral)

- Planning of wound review in 24 hours if inpatient or 48 hours if outpatient

- Consider if hand therapy required

HAND CELLULITIS

Cellulitis is acute inflammation of the skin and subcutaneous tissues. It presents as swelling and erythema to
the affected area and may or may not be associated with
a collection (Figure 3.2). Try to establish how rapidly the

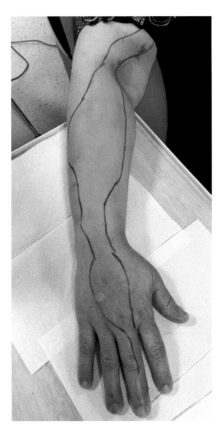

FIGURE 3.2   Cellulitis with tracking lymphangitis. This patient
required admission, IV antibiotics, elevation + close monitoring.

erythema is spreading and check for associated lymphangitis (inflammation or infection of the lymphatic system) as evidenced by red lines running up the arm. If there is a visible/palpable collection of pus, this needs to be drained as previously described (Figure 3.3). Rapid spread of cellulitis, the presence of lymphangitis, abnormal blood results or abnormal observations (e.g. fever/tachycardia) in the context of cellulitis are indications to admit for intravenous antibiotics and close monitoring.

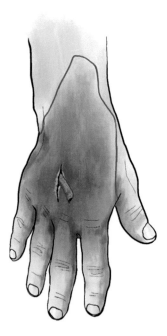

FIGURE 3.3   Insertion of trimmed inadine wick post-drainage of a collection facilitates continued drainage of the infected area. Wick can then be easily removed on ward once infection settling. Document clearly about any item placed in a wound.

If none of these are present and there is no suspicion of a collection then it may be appropriate to manage the cellulitis with oral antibiotics and monitor closely on an outpatient basis, i.e. wound review within 24–48 hours.

KEY MANAGEMENT POINTS

- Drain any collection, break loculations and leave wounds open.
- Mark and monitor extent of cellulitis.
- Treat with antibiotics and elevation.
- Patient may or may not require admission depending on severity of cellulitis.

BITE WOUNDS

Bite wounds, be they human or animal, are highly prone to infection so should be treated as infected on presentation in the emergency department. In animals the wound is generally caused by clamping of jaws around the hand/finger so remember to look volar AND dorsal to avoid missing small wounds.

Human Bites

Most human bites are 'fight bite' injuries to the hand as a result of physical confrontation. Clinicians should have a high index of suspicion in patients presenting with a laceration over the dorsum of the metacarpal phalangeal joints (MCPJ) regardless of the history. Typically, the patient has struck the mouth of the victim with a closed fist and a tooth has penetrating the skin. It is important to note that the tooth may have entered and inoculated the

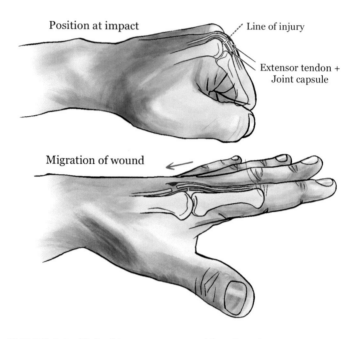

FIGURE 3.4 Fight bite at metacarpal head with inoculation of MCPJ and migration of wound when fingers extended.

underlying joint space, which will almost inevitably lead to a septic arthritis of the MCPJ (Figure 3.4). Perform X-rays as they may demonstrate a fracture or foreign body (broken tooth). Microbiology culture of these injuries typically yield *Streptococcus viridans*, *S. aureus* and *Eikenella corrodens* and are often polymicrobial with a mix of both aerobic and anaerobic organisms [i]. As the bite is commonly sustained in the clenched fist position, the skin laceration may not correspond with underlying structures if the hand is assessed with the MCPJs extended. For this reason, the wound must be assessed (and washed out) with the fingers fully flexed.

Initial management should include washing of bite wounds with iodine followed by copious saline, splinting and elevation. Though there may not yet be active signs of infection (depending on time since the injury), it is good practice to admit the patient and commence IV antibiotics. Due to the high risk of joint infection, these patients require a formal wound exploration and debridement in theatres so they should be provisionally booked on the next emergency list and discussed with a senior.

If left untreated, after a few days the area will likely become swollen, erythematous and painful. Septic arthritis, osteomyelitis and tenosynovitis are important and worryingly common sequelae of this injury. Patients presenting with active infection more than 8 days following the incident have an 18% chance of an amputation [j].

Dog Bites

Dog bites are the most common animal bite you will encounter, making up around 90% of all animal bites sustained (Figure 3.5) [k]. Like human bites they are prone to infection, with a mix of organisms that commonly include *Streptococcus* and *Staphylococcus*. As in any 'dirty' wound it is important to check the patient's tetanus status and cover them as required. If you are working in a region where rabies is endemic, it is essential to check if the animal has been vaccinated for rabies and arrange vaccination if required. Some dogs have powerful jaws so bear in mind that there may be a crush element to the injury, which may further devitalise tissue or, in the worst-case scenario, precipitate compartment syndrome.

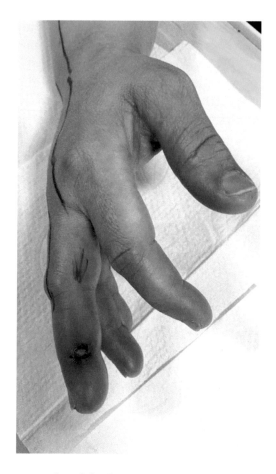

FIGURE 3.5 Infected dog bite.

All dog bites require exploration and debridement of the wound edges (either in the emergency department or more commonly in theatres), washing with iodine + saline, splinting, elevation and antibiotics. Wounds should be left open unless gaping, in which case the wound edges can be loosely approximated with Prolene sutures. It is common practice for these patients to be admitted for IV antibiotics and monitoring; however, there is no strong evidence that this is required so, depending on the centre you are working at, it may be acceptable to give oral antibiotics and review as an outpatient.

Cat Bites

Cat bites, although only responsible for 5% of animal bites, make up around 75% of those that get infected due to the long thin teeth causing puncture wounds and 'injecting' bacteria to a deep level in the tissues [k]. Infective organisms found are similar to those in dog bites with the addition of *Pasteurella multocida*. The wounds are generally small and closed on presentation in the emergency department but even if they appear uninfected (in the case of a recent bite), it is essential to debride the wound edges and irrigate the wound copiously. Wounds should be left open or ideally splinted open with an antimicrobial wick to allow free drainage of any residual infection. Again, the patient will require splinting, elevation, antibiotics and should be admitted for monitoring.

An additional consideration in cat bites is the possibility of cat scratch fever. This normally presents 3–14 days following an injury with swollen and painful lymph nodes proximal to the injury and a non-painful blister at the site of injury. It is caused by the bacteria *Bartonella henselae* in cat saliva. The disease is normally self-limiting and can be managed with simple analgesia and anti-inflammatories. In the immunocompromised there is some evidence that azithromycin can speed recovery.

KEY MANAGEMENT POINTS

- All penetrating bite wounds should be admitted for IV antibiotics and monitoring.
- Fight bites should be considered contaminated and require washout in theatres due to high incidence of associated MCPJ infection.
- Dog and cat bites should be considered contaminated and require washout either in theatres or the emergency department. Remember that the ED team see multiple bite wounds which they manage conservatively so for a referral to be made to plastics the wound is felt to be a bad one.
- Always perform X-rays.

FLEXOR SHEATH INFECTION

Infection within the flexor sheath of the digits (or flexor tenosynovitis) tend to spread along the length of the sheath and, if untreated, can destroy the delicate surfaces of the sheath and tendon leading to long-term stiffness, tendon rupture and, in the worst-case scenario, finger amputation. They account for approximately 10% of hand infections [i]. They should be considered a hand surgery emergency and treated promptly with IV antibiotics and surgical washout in theatres (*not* in the emergency department). In most, but not all, cases there is a history of sharp penetrating trauma that has breached the flexor sheath and inoculated it with bacteria. *Staphylococcus aureus* is the most common pathogen.

There are four 'Kanavel' signs of flexor sheath infection that act as the primary diagnostic tool for the condition (Table 3.2).

TABLE 3.2   Kanavel Signs of Flexor Sheath Infection

- Fusiform swelling of the digit
- Pain on passive extension
- Tenderness along the flexor sheath
- Held in semi-flexed posture

The clinical presentation can vary: Not all signs may be clinically evident. Fusiform swelling is most commonly present (Figures 3.6 and 3.7). Pain on passive extension is the most reliable sign (Figure 3.8) [1]. In addition to these

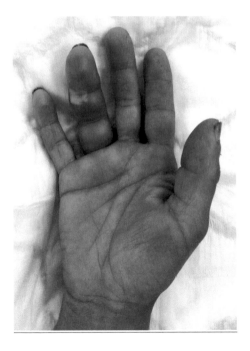

FIGURE 3.6   Flexor sheath infection of ring finger with fusiform swelling.

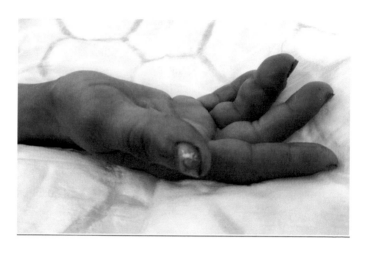

FIGURE 3.7   Finger held in semi-flexed posture.

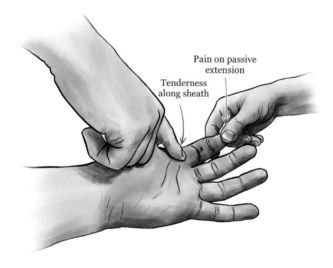

FIGURE 3.8   Examination of suspected flexor sheath infection.

signs there may be associated cellulitis. Be aware that a patient with neuropathy (most likely secondary to poorly controlled diabetes) may present late or with less convincing signs on clinical examination. Have a low threshold for getting senior input if you suspect a flexor sheath infection in this group as, should the diagnosis prove positive, the potential sequelae in terms of poor outcome or amputation is high.

Initial assessment includes a focused history and examination, bloods (including full blood count and C-reactive protein) and X-rays (to rule out the presence of a foreign body or associated fractures). Cannulas should be inserted on the UNAFFECTED side. Place the patient in a POSI splint, elevate in a Bradford sling and admit for intravenous antibiotics and washout on the emergency theatre list. Flexor sheath infections are a surgical emergency and should not wait until the following day.

If the flexor sheath infection is in the thumb or little finger be aware that the bacteria may propagate proximally and form a horseshoe abscess where the bursas communicate deep within the wrist (Parona's space) (Figure 3.9).

KEY MANAGEMENT POINTS

- Admit, consent and book for washout under GA/regional block.
- Bloods and X-ray of affected hand.
- POSI splint and elevate in Bradford sling.
- IV antibiotics and analgesia (ask ED team to put cannula on OPPOSITE side to infection).
- Make nil by mouth.

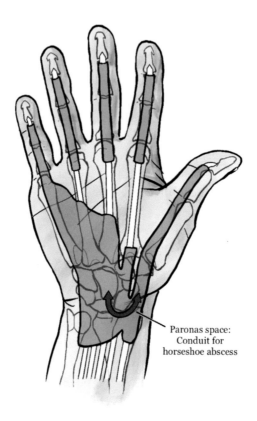

Paronas space:
Conduit for
horseshoe abscess

FIGURE 3.9 Flexor sheaths of hand. Note communication of radial and ulnar bursas in wrist.

PARONYCHIA

Paronychia is infection affecting the soft tissues surrounding the proximal or lateral nail. It is often caused by minor trauma or nail biting with *S. aureus*, the most common infective organism. It presents initially with pain, swelling

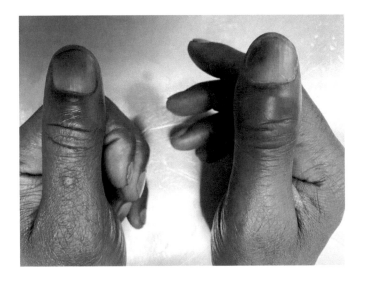

FIGURE 3.10 Paronychia of right thumb (with extension under nail). This patient required removal of nail plate.

and erythema but can progress to significant fluctuation and frank pus. Warm soaks, elevation and oral antibiotics are sufficient if there is no drainable collection. If there is evidence of fluctuance or an obvious collection of pus, incision and drainage is required, which can be performed under LA in the emergency department (Figure 3.10). Ensure any loculations are broken as you perform the drainage. Leave the incision open or consider splinting it open with a non-adherent wick. If your incision involves the nail edge, make it at an *angle* (rather than longitudinal) to the fold as this reduces the chance of devitalising this important structure (Figure 3.11). If it appears that the infection extends under the nail, then removal of the nail plate is required. X-rays should be undertaken to exclude

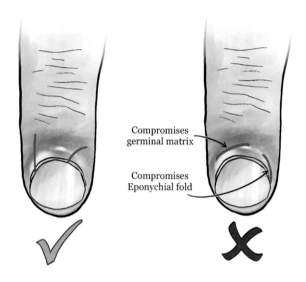

FIGURE 3.11 Good and bad incisions to drain paronychia.

early osteomyelitis, particularly if there has been recurrence of an infection or if the patient has medical risk factors. These patients do not routinely require admission and, post-drainage of the collection, can be managed with a course of oral antibiotics in the community.

KEY MANAGEMENT POINTS

- If infection involves nail bed, then the nail should be removed.
- Make incision perpendicular to nail edge to avoid devitalising eponychial fold.
- Leave wound open or splint with non-adherent gauze.
- Treat with oral antibiotics unless signs of systemic involvement.

FELON

A felon is an infection of the volar pulp of the fingertip. Longitudinal septa connect the periosteum of the distal phalanx to the skin, creating numerous fat-filled compartments in the fingertip (Figure 3.12). Normally as a result of minor trauma, infection becomes trapped in these compartments and pressure builds up. In rare cases this pressure can build to a point that compromises blood supply, which can in turn lead to tissue necrosis, septic arthritis and osteomyelitis. The most common infective organism is *S. aureus*.

Clinically, patients have an erythematous, swollen finger pulp and typically complain of a 'throbbing pain' that is exacerbated when the finger is in a dependent position. X-rays should be performed to check for any residual foreign body or evidence of early osteomyelitis.

Incision and drainage can be performed under LA in the emergency department. Make a longitudinal incision over the area of maximum fluctuance and ensure all involved septa are disrupted by probing the infected area

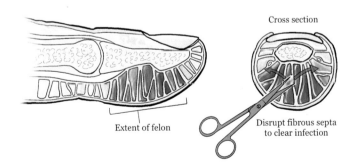

Cross section

Extent of felon

Disrupt fibrous septa to clear infection

FIGURE 3.12   Anatomy of finger pulp + felon infection.

with a semi-sharp instrument like the tip of a plastic forceps, followed by washout with iodine and copious saline. Splint the incision open with a wick to allow the infection to continue to drain.

With the addition of oral antibiotics, these patients rarely require admission, but should be closely followed up in 24–48 hours for a dressing change and wound check. The wound can be left to heal by secondary intention.

CHAPTER 4

Hand Trauma – Soft Tissue

Hand trauma will form the majority of the referrals you receive on call. Though the nature and treatment of injuries vary widely, the initial management steps are similar in all cases: Wound irrigation and control of bleeding, splinting and elevation, tetanus and antibiotics. The main decisions you have to make is whether a patient requires admission to the hospital and whether they require an operation. If they do require an operation, the next decision will be: How soon and via what pathway?

BLEEDING

Almost all bleeding, including arterial bleeding, can be controlled with direct pressure, elevation and patience. Often when you attend a patient in resus who has a severed ulnar or radial artery a tight tourniquet style dressing has been applied

DOI: 10.1201/9781003163770-4

to the forearm and, as a result, the hand is cold. Prepare your dressings and then carefully remove the tourniquet. If there is time (and with the patient's permission), obtain a photograph of the injury as this may aid operative planning. If the bleeding has stopped or is an ooze this is likely because it is stemmed by formation of a haematoma in the wound. Do NOT remove this haematoma. Elevate the limb and observe the hand to check that it reperfuses. If when you remove the tourniquet there IS arterial bleeding, apply point pressure with gauze to identify where to stem it. Once you have identified the bleeding source then quickly remove the gauze and pack with a coagulation promoting interface (Kaltostat, Aquacel or Celox) followed by lots of rolled up gauze. Push it right into the wound if need be. Again, apply pressure, elevate and observe for a few minutes to see if bleeding is stemmed and hand remaining perfused (via the other artery). You can then apply more folded gauze or a roll of crepe to maintain the point pressure you have been exerting with your fingers. If you can do this in a targeted way you can then bandage the arm without compromising the flow of the other artery (Figure 4.1). Managed in this way, operative repair can take place on the next emergency day-time list rather than out of hours. Note: Arterial injuries are often associated with nerve injuries.

If you are unsuccessful, or if you suspect division of both ulnar and radial arteries reapply the tourniquet and contact your registrar immediately.

NAILBED INJURIES

The nail plate grows from the fold of germinal matrix proximally so, as long as this germinal matrix is largely undamaged, the nail plate can be removed to facilitate repair of

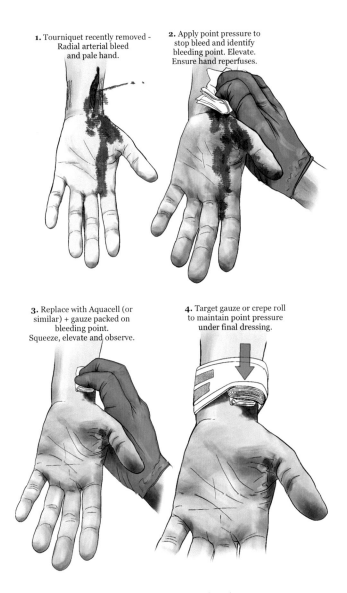

1. Tourniquet recently removed - Radial arterial bleed and pale hand.

2. Apply point pressure to stop bleed and identify bleeding point. Elevate. Ensure hand reperfuses.

3. Replace with Aquacell (or similar) + gauze packed on bleeding point. Squeeze, elevate and observe.

4. Target gauze or crepe roll to maintain point pressure under final dressing.

FIGURE 4.1   Forearm bleeding control technique.

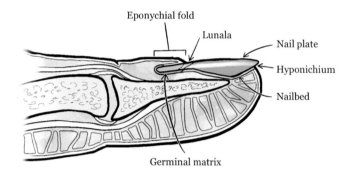

FIGURE 4.2   Anatomy of nailbed.

the underlying nailbed in the expectation that the nail will regrow (Figure 4.2). Injuries to the nailbed can lead to irregular nail growth and infection of the underlying tissues. There is not much tissue between the nail plate and the dorsal aspect of the distal phalanx so there is potential for bacterial colonisation of the bone if the nail plate is damaged and a thorough washout is not performed. Nailbed repairs can be carried out in the emergency department or trauma clinic under LA and, as such, are a common on-call task.

Nailbed injuries are often associated with underlying tuft fractures of the distal phalanx. These do not generally need fixation. However, if the fracture involves the mid or proximal aspect of the phalanx and the fragment is displaced the patient may require a formal procedure with K-wire stabilisation. That said, if the nailbed requires repair under local anaesthetic, you will need to washout the fracture site anyway and, through manipulation and a sound repair of the skin/nailbed, one can often reduce the fracture at the same time as repairing the nailbed. Perform a repeat X-ray post-nailbed repair and if the reduction is acceptable, you will have saved the patient a formal procedure. You can then simply zimmer splint the finger (on the volar aspect) and follow up the fracture as an outpatient (further information in *Fractures and dislocations* chapter).

When consenting for a nailbed repair advise that initial nail regrowth may be uneven looking but that it will improve over 6–9 months. Warn that the nail may always appear abnormal. Other risks to mention are: Stiffness, cold intolerance and altered sensation.

Nailbed injuries are very common in children, with the normal mechanism of injury being a crush in a door (Figure 4.3). Remember to check the tetanus status of your

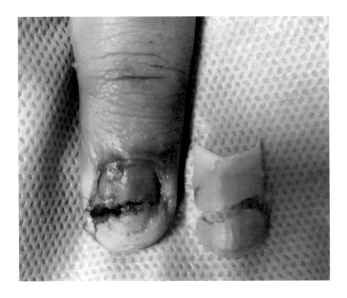

FIGURE 4.3   Simple nailbed injury pre-repair of nailbed.

patient and offer tetanus if they are not up to date. If the wound is dirty offer antibiotics. In adults and older children, the repair can be carried out under a simple ring block. In younger children either ketamine sedation or GA is required.

When assessing the injury be aware that an intact nail does not mean the underlying nailbed is intact. If there is an underlying tuft fracture, greater than 50% subungual haematoma, or partial avulsion of the nail plate, it is best to remove the nail plate to assess and repair the nailbed.

Injuries range from minor damage of the nailbed to almost complete amputation of the tip (Figure 4.4). The

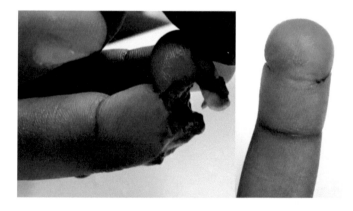

FIGURE 4.4   Nailbed + partial tip amputation in a child. Despite the relatively small volar skin bridge the tip remained perfused and only repair of the skin laterally + nailbed repair was required in this patient.

latter is common in children who sustain a severe crush injury in a door. Don't panic! Only a small volar tissue bridge is required for the partially amputated tip to remain perfused so check CRT as it may well be normal. Carry out your repair in the same way. It is optimal to perform nailbed repairs (especially in children) with the assistance of loupes.

Nailbed Repair Technique

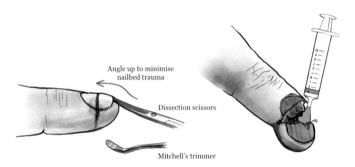

FIGURE 4.5A   Once the local anaesthetic has taken effect, apply a finger tourniquet and remove the nail.* A Mitchells trimmer is ideal for this, though dissecting scissors are also suitable. *As you slide your instrument under the nail direct its sharp tip slightly upwards to minimise trauma to the nailbed.* Once partially mobilised, the nail plate can be rolled off with a needle holder. Wash the wound thoroughly and remove any haematoma.

---

* *Note:* In some centres you may be advised to use LA with adrenaline and no tourniquet, particularly in paediatric patients. This means there is no reactive bleeding when the tourniquet comes down causing bleeding into the dressing and painful dressing changes down the line as the blood dries.

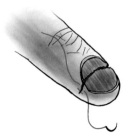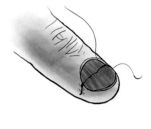

FIGURE 4.5B   If the tip is partially amputated start by repairing the (non-nailbed) skin laterally with a 4-0 or 5-0 absorbable suture. Then repair the nailbed with a 6-0-gauge absorbable suture. Apply only gentle tension to the nailbed sutures and only pull the suture material through in the direction of your suture bite, as it is easy for the suture to cut through the nailbed causing further damage.

Once the repair is complete apply a non-adherent interface such as Mepitel or Adaptic touch and a conventional dressing (gauze, crepe, tape). Some seniors advocate cleaning and replacing the nail to splint the nailbed flat; however, this may increase the risk of infection [m]. Elevate the finger, and gently squeeze it and then remove the finger tourniquet to minimise initial bleeding as the finger reperfuses. These patients require a wound check and change of dressing by a nurse in 4–5 days (outpatient or in the community) but do not normally require follow-up by the plastics team. In paediatric patients you may choose to bring them back to a plastics dressing clinic for their wound check after a slightly longer time frame (up to 14 days) as it is less painful and distressing to change the dressing after a delay.

KEY MANAGEMENT POINTS

- Obtain X-rays.
- Ensure up to date with tetanus.
- Repair lateral (non-nailbed) tissue, then repair the nailbed.
- Be aware of Seymour fracture pattern in paediatric patients.

Seymour Fracture (in Children)

This is a displaced transverse fracture across the growth plate of the distal phalanx in association with a nailbed injury (Figures 4.6, 4.7 and 4.8). It is important to be aware of this injury pattern as the child will require a formal procedure in theatres to reduce and pin the fracture rather than the simple nailbed repair that can be offered in ED.

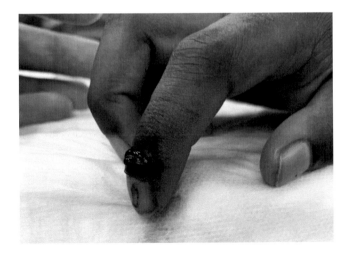

FIGURE 4.6 Seymour fracture presentation.

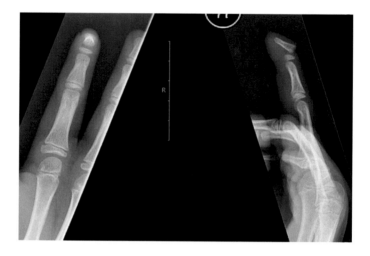

FIGURE 4.7 Seymour fracture X-ray (same patient as pictured).

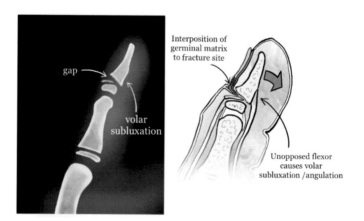

FIGURE 4.8 Anatomy of Seymour fracture.

This is due to two factors: (1) There may be interposition of soft tissue at the fracture site (often the germinal matrix), which prevents reduction of the fracture. (2) As the extensor tendon inserts into the epiphysis but the flexor inserts more distally into the metaphysis, there is an unopposed flexion force on the distal fragment, which prevents it returning to its anatomical position. Clinical presentation is of a mallet finger with associated nailbed injury.

DISTAL TIP AMPUTATION

These injuries are not only commonly sustained as a result of knife accidents preparing food but also occur in children as part of nailbed injuries (Figure 4.9). A useful rule of thumb is: *If there is no bone exposed it is best to let the wound heal by secondary intention.* If you are not sure if bone is exposed then put in a LA ring block, apply a finger tourniquet and clean the wound. Press with an instrument to see if you get the hard 'tap' feedback of exposed bone. If the bone is only slightly exposed you can put in a couple of dissolvable

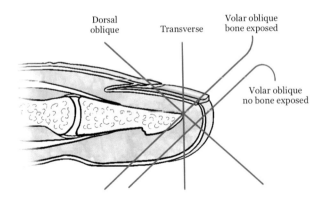

FIGURE 4.9   Anatomy of distal fingertip injuries.

sutures to approximate the (open) soft tissue over the bone in the hope of allowing it to heal by secondary intention. Apply a non-adherent dressing and follow up these patients in a dressings clinic ± outpatient clinic within 4–5 days to assess healing. In most cases they have a good functional outcome, regaining sensation as the skin heals, albeit with an altered contour to the end of the finger and possibly a shortened nail.

If the bone is fully exposed the patient will require a terminalisation or reconstructive procedure to achieve soft tissue coverage. The decision between terminalisation and reconstruction is influenced by a number of factors including age, patient preference, severity of injury, hand dominance, occupation and comorbid medical conditions. Liaise with your senior to plan the appropriate procedure, normally carried out as an emergency outpatient procedure.

If the patient has brought in an amputated tip AND the bone is exposed AND the mechanism of injury is clean AND it occurred within the last 4–6 hours you can consider suturing the amputated tissue back on as a composite graft. This procedure has a higher chance of success in paediatric than in adult patients [n]. Check with your registrar on a case-by-case basis before attempting a composite graft. It is important to advise the patient that there is a significant chance that the graft will not take and, even if it does take, they will likely experience reduced sensation in the area. The advantage of attempting the composite graft is an improved contour to the finger. Even if the graft does not take (becomes black and ultimately falls off) it can function as a temporising biological dressing and provide a good environment for granulation tissue to grow over the bone tip which may mean the patient avoids terminalisation/reconstruction of the finger.

KEY MANAGEMENT POINTS

- If no bone exposed, leave to heal by secondary intention.
- If bone is exposed, liaise with your senior as to appropriate surgical management, plan on a case-by-case basis.
- Ensure patient is up to date with tetanus and consider antibiotics if any concern of wound contamination.

TENDON INJURIES

Tendon injuries are common, making up a large proportion of the on-call workload. It is important to diagnose and treat them early as primary repair becomes more difficult with time, due to the proximal end retracting and shortening. This is more the case with flexor tendons as extensor tendons have junctura tendineae which reduce retraction. Tendons should ideally be repaired within 4 days of injury, and 2 weeks is generally considered the maximum time period where primary repair may still be possible. Thereafter, the patient will likely require a 2-stage repair or a tendon transfer. Unless multiple flexors are divided (spaghetti wrist or large palm laceration), patients with tendon injuries do not need to be admitted and can be brought in as emergency day case procedures.

Tendon injuries are commonly caused by sharp penetrating trauma such as a knife or broken glass. The entry wound may be small. A finger that cannot be flexed at all and is held in fixed extension is a giveaway for complete division of both flexor digitorum profundus (FDP) and flexor digitorum superficialis (FDS)

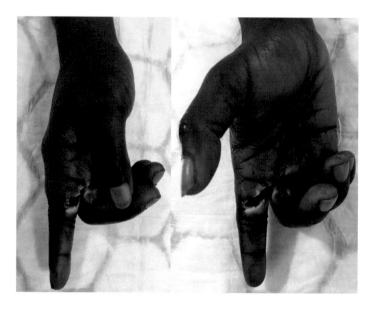

FIGURE 4.10   Clinically 100% division of FDS and FDP of index finger, Zone 2 injury. Note complete loss of the natural cascade of the index finger.

tendons (Figure 4.10). Isolated damage to one flexor tendon may be discernible on clinical examination of the individual tendons – see the chapter on Hand Assessment.

The extensor mechanism is complex, which can result in patients retaining function even when there is significant tendon damage. If there is a wound at the PIPJ, it is important to perform Elson's test to assess if there is a central slip injury (Figure 4.11).

In a more proximal partial extensor tendon injury, the patient may still retain good extension due to the spread of the extensor hood.

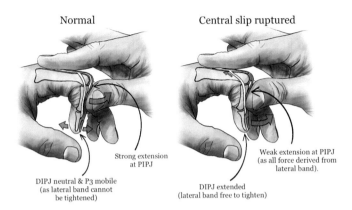

Normal   Central slip ruptured

Strong extension
at PIPJ

Weak extension at PIPJ
(as all force derived from
lateral band).

DIPJ neutral & P3 mobile
(as lateral band cannot
be tightened)

DIPJ extended
(lateral band free to tighten)

FIGURE 4.11   Elson's test for central slip integrity. Hold the PIPJ in full flexion then ask the patient to extend their distal phalanx. If central slip is intact they *cannot* extend the DIPJ, if central slip ruptured they *are able to extend*.

Damage to tendons where a movement is driven by more than one tendon (such as wrist flexion) is hard to gauge so bear this in mind when deciding your degree of suspicion of tendon damage.

It is important to include assessment of the neurovascular status of the digit distal to the injury, particularly if both flexor tendons have been divided, as it may be the case that the volar neurovascular bundles have also been affected. If just one neurovascular bundle has been divided the finger should be sensate on the opposite side and well perfused. *If you are concerned that both neurovascular bundles have been divided, i.e. numbness on both sides of the digit, the patient will need urgent senior review as they may require a revascularisation to save the digit.*

In a similar manner if there is a flexor tendon injury in the proximal palm there is a higher degree of urgency for exploration and repair as here the tendons lie deep to the superficial palmar arch and if this is damaged the patient will benefit from a revascularisation of this structure.

Sometimes a tendon is partially cut. In this instance the patient may report some weakness/pain on flexion/extension or the examination may be normal. A partial tendon injury warrants exploration ± repair as there is a risk that the tendon will rupture in the future. It is therefore important to take the time to examine the wound under local anaesthetic as without analgesia one can either miss tendon damage (especially if partial) or unnecessarily book the patient for a formal procedure when in fact the wound has not breached any tendons or significant structures. In partial tendon damage the section of the tendon that is damaged may not be immediately visible as their hand may have been in a different position at the time of injury. Therefore, *move* the affected finger/hand as you look at the gliding tendon in the wound bed to bring the damaged section into view. Remember to always assess for associated nerve injury before putting in local anaesthetic. Document the zone of injury in your findings as this will assist the surgeon planning the procedure (Figures 4.12 and 4.13).

Less common than open injuries to tendons are closed flexor tendon ruptures. These occur by a sudden pull against the tendon when the patient is gripping something, often when playing contact sport: 'rugby jersey injury'. In the case of a tendon rupture the patient may report the sensation of feeling the tendon suddenly 'go' and on examination function is completely absent. Generally, the injury will have occurred at the insertion of the tendon. These patients require a formal Zone 1 tendon repair with a Mitek bone anchor.

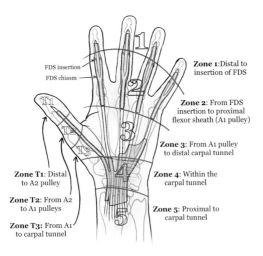

FIGURE 4.12   Flexor tendon zones.

Patients with (open) tendon injuries require washing and dressing of the wounds, a POSI splint and a sling while awaiting operative repair. Ensure tetanus is up to date and unless the mechanism of injury and wound are very clean and the patient has no medical risk factors, prescribe oral antibiotics.

As flexor tendons are deep structures, with the potential to significantly retract and which require a more complex repair technique, consent these patients for the procedure under GA or regional block as per your centres policy. A single-digit extensor repair can normally be done under LA but if there are multiple extensors cut or the thumb is involved then GA/regional anaesthetic may be more prudent. When consenting, advise the patient they will have to wear a splint afterwards, will need physiotherapy and will not be able to use their hand normally for up to 3 months. Advise that smoking can significantly affect tendon healing.

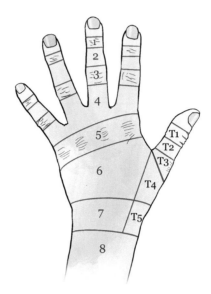

FIGURE 4.13   Extensor tendon zones. Remember that the odd numbers are over joints.

KEY MANAGEMENT POINTS

- Suspect tendon injury in stabbing injuries with sharp objects.
- If you are not sure if a tendon is damaged, take the time to examine the wound under LA. If you are still not sure then book for a formal examination under anaesthesia.
- Consent flexor tendon repairs under GA or regional block. Single extensors can be done under LA.
- If a tendon injury is more than 2 weeks old it will likely need reconstruction – discuss with a senior.
- Ensure patient up to date with tetanus and prescribe oral antibiotics while awaiting surgery.

NERVE INJURIES

Divided nerves (neurotmesis) require urgent formal surgical repair under magnification within 4 days of injury for digital nerves [o] or within 3 days for major nerves of the upper limb. Digital nerves can be repaired on an outpatient basis. Patients with major nerve injuries should be admitted and managed as inpatients. If left unrepaired for any significant time nerves retract, making primary repair difficult. Neuroma may also occur.

Digital nerve injuries secondary to sharp penetrating trauma can be isolated or occur in conjunction with tendon injuries. If not repaired they affect long-term function particularly if they involve the thumb or leading edges of the hand, i.e. ulnar aspect of little finger or radial aspect of index finger. Because of the close anatomical relationship between the digital nerve and digital artery, it is generally the case that if the patient has numbness on one side of a finger, then the artery on that side is divided. Equally, if there is an arterial bleed from one side of a finger, you can be confident that the associated digital nerve is divided.

Ask the patient if they noticed numbness *immediately* after the injury. If they did; it is highly suggestive of nerve division. Partial numbness that evolves slowly after an injury may be due to pressure on an undamaged nerve from swelling or bleeding. An important anatomical variation to note is that in the thumb the volar neurovascular bundles lie much closer to the midline of the digit than in the fingers. In the palm there may be damage to a common digital nerve affecting the radial border of one finger and the ulnar border of another.

Because digital nerves are small, it is hard to assess if they are damaged by looking into the wound under local anaesthetic. Your decision as to whether to book the patient for formal exploration and nerve repair is, therefore, guided by the degree of numbness and the importance of the nerve (e.g. have a lower threshold for exploration if area is on a leading edge of the hand).

Assessment of damage to the Ulnar nerve, Median nerve and superficial branch of the Radial nerve due to more proximal penetrating trauma is as per the steps and anatomy described in Hand Assessment chapter. Bear in mind the likelihood of associated injuries due to the close anatomical relationships between: (1) the Median nerve and flexor tendons to the digits + palmaris longus tendon (2) the Ulnar nerve and the Ulnar artery + FCU tendon. If damage to the Median or Ulnar nerve is suspected admit the patient and discuss the case urgently with a senior.

Initial management for an isolated digital nerve injury is again that of washing, dressing, checking of tetanus status and oral antibiotics (if required). If a major nerve is injured the patient will additionally need splinting in a POSI while they await surgery.

KEY MANAGEMENT POINTS

- Digital nerves can be repaired as emergency day case procedures. Major nerves require admission for repair within 3 days.
- Nerve injuries often occur in conjunction with tendon injuries.
- If patient reports numbness immediately after injury, nerve damage is very likely.
- Ensure tetanus status is up to date and consider antibiotics.

MALLET FINGER

A mallet finger is an injury to the extensor mechanism at the level of the DIPJ. Patients present with the DIPJ held in flexion due to the (newly unopposed) force exerted by the FDP tendon.

The injury may be closed or open. Closed injuries are most common and generally occur when there has been sudden forced flexion at the DIPJ causing avulsion of the extensor tendon at its insertion into the distal phalanx. On X-ray there may be nothing to see; there may be a small avulsion fracture from the site of the tendon insertion, or there may be a significant dorsal avulsion fragment with associated volar subluxation of the distal phalanx. An open injury may be a simple transverse laceration which has divided the extensor (no bony injury) or there may be a deep abrasion with loss of skin/tendon substance and exposed bone.

Closed Mallet

If there is no bony avulsion on X-ray put the patient in a zimmer splint with the DIPJ joint hyperextended and refer to hand therapy (or plastics outpatient – as per your local guidelines) (Figure 4.14). Healing will take place by the tendon scarring down to its insertion. Advise the patient they must *not* remove the splint for the period advised (usually 6 weeks) as this will reavulse the tendon and reset the clock in terms of the healing process. Follow-up can be managed by the hand therapy team.

If there is a bony avulsion <1/3 of the DIPJ articular surface and there is no associated volar subluxation of the distal phalanx, again splint the joint in hyperextension

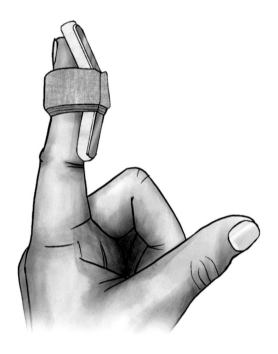

FIGURE 4.14 Hyperextension splint for management of closed mallet finger.

and re-X-ray. If the reduction of the fracture is good and the patient compliant it can be managed conservatively by strict splinting and monitoring under the hand therapy team. If the fracture will not reduce book the patient for reduction and K-wire fixation under LA (Figure 4.15).

If there is bony avulsion >1/3 of the DIPJ articular surface AND/OR there is associated volar subluxation of the distal phalanx the patient will require emergency day case surgery. Book them for reduction and K-wire fixation

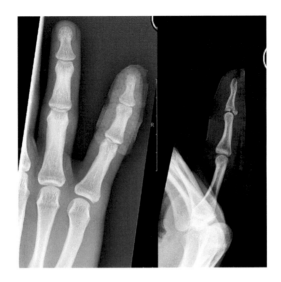

FIGURE 4.15   Closed bony mallet with adequate fracture congruity for bony healing. Despite the fracture involving >1/3 of articular surface this patient was successfully managed conservatively with a hyperextension Zimmer splint.

under LA and splint them in hyperextension while they await this (Figure 4.16).

Open Mallet

Simple transverse lacerations with minimal associated tissue loss should be booked for primary repair under LA on a designated emergency day case list.

Open injuries with significant soft tissue or tendon loss should be booked for repair ± local flap reconstruction ± tendon graft under regional or general anaesthetic on a designated emergency day case list when a senior registrar or consultant is present.

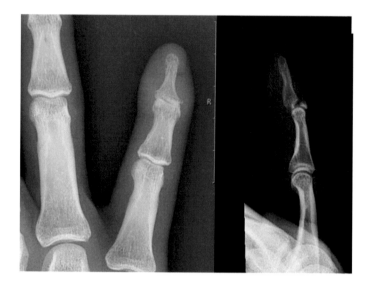

FIGURE 4.16   Closed bony mallet involving >1/3 of articular surface and volar subluxation of P3 + no congruity of fracture site. This patient required operative reduction and K-wire stabilisation.

KEY MANAGEMENT POINTS

- Closed mallet injury with no bony involvement = hyperextension splint and refer to HT.

FOREIGN BODIES

Foreign bodies in the finger or hand are common referrals. Metal (e.g. a sewing or hypodermic needle) is easily visible on X-ray, glass is less clear but normally visible, wood and plastic are rarely visible. Fish spines and palm fronds can be particularly irritant. In your history take note of how long ago the foreign body went in. Generally, patients will present acutely with pain ± infection, but if they are presenting with symptoms, a number of weeks down the line then scar tissue will have formed around the foreign body making its location and removal much more challenging. In this group it is not advisable to attempt removal in ED.

If the foreign body is large/causing significant pain/infected then it should be removed. Occasionally, particularly in a late presentation with a healed wound, minor symptoms and a small foreign body you can counsel the patient that it is acceptable to leave it, as an attempt at removal may not be successful and may also cause new symptoms due to the surgical exploration.

Depending on the size and location of the foreign body, and especially if it is easily palpable, you may be able to remove it in under LA in the emergency department. If it is glass or plastic ask the patient what colour it is as this may help you see it. Counsel the patient that you may not be successful, but that if you do succeed, it will save them coming back for a formal procedure on another occasion. Obtain X-rays and carefully correlate these with the patient's finger marking out where you think the object is. After numbing the finger and applying a tourniquet make a longitudinal cut over the suspected location of the object and probe to sense the feedback when your instrument strikes the foreign body. Remove with forceps or a needle holder and (if there are no signs of infection) close the wound. Perform a repeat X-ray post-removal to confirm there are no residual foreign bodies remaining. If you are not successful bring them back for removal on a formal list where X-ray will be available. Prescribe tetanus/antibiotics as appropriate. If there is no functional deficit they do not require follow-up.

KEY MANAGEMENT POINTS

- If foreign body is superficial + easily visible on X-ray + a significant size it can likely be removed under local anaesthetic in ED.
- If foreign body has been embedded for a number of weeks do not attempt removal in ED.

CHAPTER 5

Hand Trauma – Fractures and Dislocations

The general principle in management of all fractures is to strike the optimal balance between allowing the patient to mobilise as early as possible (to avoid stiffness and deconditioning) whilst protecting the fracture site so it can safely heal.

At one end of this spectrum lies inherently stable minor fractures, which require no immobilisation, at the other end of the spectrum are complex fractures which require an extended period of immobilisation (by splinting or by surgical fixation) to allow bone healing before mobilising.

Key points in the history include date fracture sustained, mechanism of injury, hand dominance and occupation. Ask the referring team to obtain three views of the fracture site (AP, oblique and lateral) if they have not already done so. Ask if there is scissoring or deformity of the finger/hand but know that you need to see the patient in person to properly assess this. If the patient is a smoker, inform them that the main way they can avoid non-union of their fracture is to stop smoking.

Displaced fractures are described according to the position of the distal part in relation to the proximal part. The Salter-Harris classification is only used with paediatric fractures.

CLOSED FRACTURES GENERAL PRINCIPLES

Closed fractures of the hand require (1) examination and (2) imaging to enable you to decide whether operative or conservative management is appropriate. If operative management is required, it can be arranged on an urgent outpatient basis.

The only caveat to this is when there are multiple closed fractures or if you have a concern such as impending compartment syndrome due to a crush injury – in these scenarios, the patient needs to be admitted.

If the fracture position is acceptable on X-ray AND the patient does not have significant deformity on examination, closed fractures can be splinted in plaster or buddy taped and followed up a week as an outpatient to confirm that the fracture position has not worsened. The reason for 1 week follow-up is that in this timeframe the fracture will remain mobile, so if it slips, the operation can still be done under favourable conditions.

If the fracture position is non-acceptable on X-ray AND/OR the patient has significant deformity on examination, they will require an intervention. Some fractures are amenable to manipulation under local anaesthetic (MUA) in the ED/trauma clinic setting. When this works it is an excellent management pathway as the patient is saved a return for a formal procedure. Unless you have had tuition you will not be expected to perform MUAs at the start of your plastics rotation, but it is useful to build these skills so take every opportunity to learn. If the fracture pattern is not amenable to an MUA OR the MUA is unsuccessful (X-ray or examination still unacceptable) then book the patient for a formal fracture fixation.

OPEN FRACTURES GENERAL PRINCIPLES

Open fractures, once assessed with imaging and clinical examination, should always be admitted and managed operatively with a formal washout $\pm$ fracture fixation.

This is in addition to IV antibiotics and tetanus prophylaxis. If you review a patient who has an open wound + a fracture but you are not convinced the wound communicates with the fracture site seek senior input or, to be on the safe side, admit the patient. It is better to be mildly reprimanded for a soft admission than the more serious consequences of sending an open fracture home.

Fractures of Finger Metacarpals

Metacarpal fractures are generally caused by punching a hard object or from an impact to the dorsum of the hand. The most common fracture sites of the metacarpal are neck and shaft, with fractures to the base and head less common. The most common fracture you will encounter is a closed 'boxers fracture', which is a fracture to the neck of the 5th metacarpal.

Neck Fractures

Neck fractures commonly heal unless they are completely off ended (Figures 5.1 and 5.2). As long as there is minimal extensor lag and no rotational deformity, then a significant degree of volar angulation at the fracture site is acceptable and a large proportion of these fractures can be managed conservatively ± an MUA (Figure 5.3). A greater degree of angulation deformity is acceptable in the 5th metacarpal than in the 4th to 2nd metacarpals. If managing a neck fracture conservatively put the patient in a volar POSI splint (or ulnar gutter if 5th metacarpal) and counsel them that their knuckle may appear depressed long term but that they should not suffer a functional deficit.

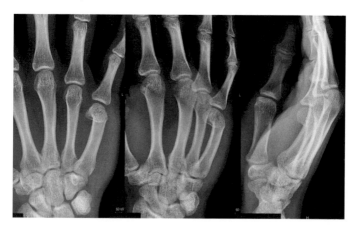

FIGURE 5.1   Fifth metacarpal neck 'boxers' fracture for conservative management. This patient had no rotation or extensor lag and the angulation of the fracture is acceptable.

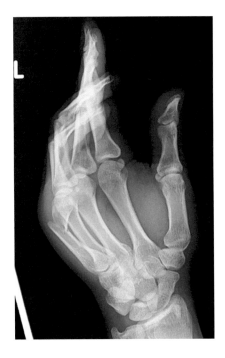

FIGURE 5.2 Metacarpal neck (Boxers) fracture for operative management. This patient had a significant extensor lag and the fracture position was not improved by an MUA.

Indications for intervention [p]

- Significant angulation deformity
- Off ended on X-ray
- Rotational deformity/scissoring
- Extensor lag
- Shortening >3 mm (compare with other side)

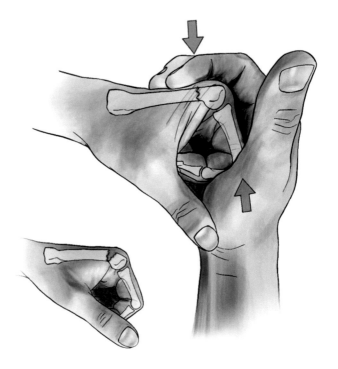

FIGURE 5.3   JAHSS manoeuvre – a common MUA technique for metacarpal neck fracture. Flex the PIPJ and apply pressure as above to reduce the fracture.

Shaft Fractures

Shaft fractures can be classified as transverse, oblique or spiral. Transverse fractures are normally caused by an axial load (such as a fall or a punch), whereas spiral and oblique fractures are caused by torsional forces. The majority of shaft fractures are stable and can be managed conservatively (Figures 5.4 and 5.5). Fractures to the 3rd and 4th metacarpal shafts are inherently more stable than the 2nd and

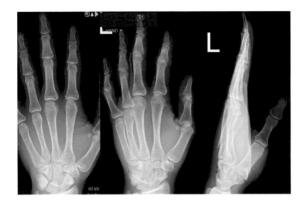

FIGURE 5.4   Oblique (butterfly) midshaft fracture with minimally displaced dorsal spike. As this fracture was minimally displaced, it was managed conservatively.

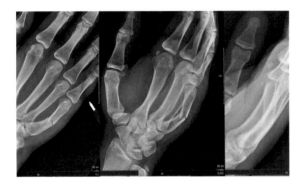

FIGURE 5.5   Transverse midshaft fracture with approximately 30 degrees of volar angulation. This can be managed conservatively or operatively. MUA + conservative management in a cast has the advantage of no tissue disruption but a significant period of immobilisation. Open reduction and plate fixation has the advantage of early mobilisation but involves disruption to tissues and small risks associated with an operation.

5th as they are flanked on both sides by stabilising tissue. MUA can often be successful in bringing the fracture to an acceptable position for conservative management. After performing the MUA apply a POSI volar or dorsal blocking splint before re-X-raying the patient to reassess the fracture. If the reduction is satisfactory then arrange follow-up in a hand clinic according to your locally agreed protocol.

Indications for intervention [p]:

- Rotational deformity/scissoring
- Significant angulation at fracture site
- Significant displacement on X-ray
- Shortening >3 mm (compare with other side)

Head Fractures

Head fractures are rare, usually resulting from axial loading or dislocation at the MCPJ. In the context of a punch injury with a laceration and head fracture the joint capsule will have been breached and the patient will require a formal washout ± fracture fixation. In closed fractures, if less than 20% of the articular surface is involved AND there is less than 1 mm articular step-off AND the fracture is not grossly displaced then conservative management is appropriate (Figure 5.6).

Indications for intervention [p]

- >1 mm of articular step-off
- >25% of articular surface involved
- Significant displacement

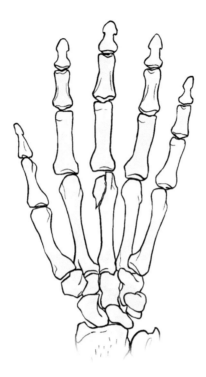

FIGURE 5.6 Fracture of metacarpal head. As there is >1 mm articular step off + >25% of articular surface involved and the fracture is non-comminuted this should be managed surgically.

- Scissoring on examination
- Non-comminuted fracture amenable to headless screws

Base Fractures

Metacarpal base fractures usually occur from axial load (punch or fall) when the wrist is flexed volarly. These fractures are sometimes associated with carpometacarpal dislocation which, if present, requires senior review and early reduction. Assess the lateral X-ray carefully as what appears acceptable on AP and oblique may demonstrate significant dorsal displacement (or dislocation) on the lateral view (Figure 5.7). If the fracture pattern appears complex or unclear consider booking the patient for a CT hand/wrist.

Indications for intervention [p]

- Significant displacement of fracture

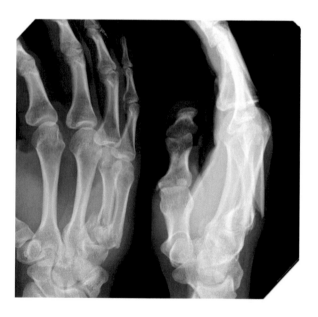

FIGURE 5.7   Significantly displaced and impacted short oblique fractures of 4th and 5th metacarpal bases. No dislocation at MCPJs. Due to the displacement these fractures were managed surgically with closed reduction and K-wire stabilisation.

Fractures of Thumb Metacarpal Base

Fractures of the thumb metacarpal base behave differently to the finger metacarpals due to the forces of the tendons inserting on the bone.

A Bennett fracture is a two-part unstable intra-articular fracture at the base of the thumb metacarpal. The ulnar fragment remains held in place by the volar beak ligament and the metacarpal subluxes proximally (due to the force of abductor pollicis longus) and rotates towards supination (due to the forces of adductor pollicis and flexor pollicis brevis) (Figure 5.8).

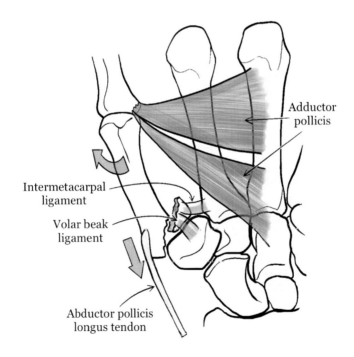

FIGURE 5.8   Bennetts fracture anatomy.

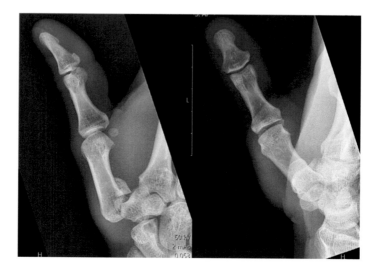

FIGURE 5.9   Bennetts fracture requiring surgical reduction and K-wire stabilisation.

Management of these fractures is almost always operative due to the inherent instability of the fracture pattern and the high (potential) morbidity of a non-healed thumb fracture. Reduction of the fracture is achieved by firm abduction and pronation of the thumb whilst applying pressure to the radial base of the metacarpal (Figure 5.9).

A Rolando fracture is any comminuted intraarticular fracture of the thumb metacarpal base (Figure 5.10). For the same reasons these are usually managed operatively by K-wire or plate fixation.

Fractures of Proximal and Middle Phalanx

Causes of fractures to the phalanxes vary widely and include crush, twisting and axial forces. The PIPJ has a

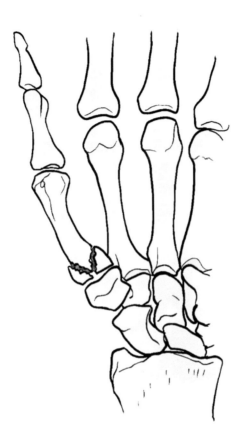

FIGURE 5.10   Rolando fracture pattern.

large arc of movement of up to 110 degrees so fractures affecting this joint have the potential to significantly affect long-term function of the finger. Particularly problematic is the pilon or 'burst' fracture at the base of P2 (sustained by sudden axial load), which is surgically challenging to reduce and repair. Fractures affecting the DIPJ, even if severe, do not cause the same morbidity.

Phalangeal Base Fractures

In children the most common hand fracture is a Salter-Harris 2 fracture at the base of the proximal phalanx, often to the little finger (Figure 5.11). The incidence of this fracture increases from around age 10 as children become more involved in active sport. If the fracture is undisplaced or minimally displaced on X-ray AND there is no deformity on examination the finger can be buddy strapped to its neighbour. The child can mobilise gently and be followed

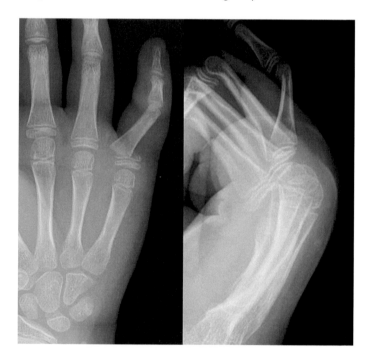

FIGURE 5.11   Salter Harris 2 displaced fracture at base of P1. This required MUA under GA.

up as an outpatient with an X-ray in 1 week to check the fracture position.

If there is significant angulation on X-ray OR deformity on examination an intervention is required. These fractures can generally be treated with an MUA. Ideally this is done in clinic/ED under LA ± Entonox but if they will not tolerate this, they will need to be booked to have it under GA. In rare cases where the fracture is unstable K-wire stabilisation may be required, so if they are coming in for a formal procedure add this to the consent form. As a rule of thumb: Insertion of metalwork in paediatric fractures is avoided where possible.

In adults, base of P2 fractures occurs as pilon fractures from a sudden axial load to the finger (Figure 5.12). Unless the displacement is minimal these often require application of a surgical traction device to reduce ± K-wire fixation of the fracture fragments. Seek senior input in planning management as there is high morbidity associated with handling this fracture pattern poorly.

Shaft Fractures

Minimally displaced fractures of the phalangeal shaft may be amenable to conservative management (Figure 5.13). Transverse or short oblique fractures, if in a good position on X-ray AND no deformity on examination, are less likely to slip so can be put in a volar POSI splint and followed up in 1 week with a check X-ray. Long oblique and spiral fractures are more unstable and given to rotational deformity, so have a much lower threshold to book these for surgical

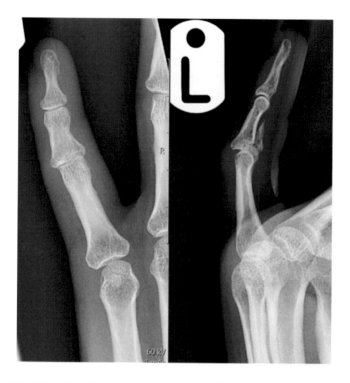

FIGURE 5.12   Pilon fracture to base of P2. Note loss of joint space and comminution of fracture making this very difficult to manage surgically. This required an external traction device (Suzuki frame).

fixation (Figure 5.14). Fixation is commonly with percutaneous crossed K-wires though plates or screws may sometimes be used.

Neck Fractures

Phalangeal neck fractures are very rare in adults but more common in children. If minimally displaced and no

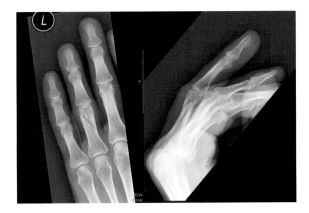

FIGURE 5.13 Minimally displaced oblique P1 fracture. This was managed conservatively in a POSI splint. Close surveillance was required as this fracture pattern is not stable.

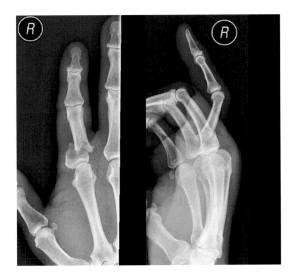

FIGURE 5.14 Significantly displaced transverse shaft fracture requiring open reduction and internal fixation.

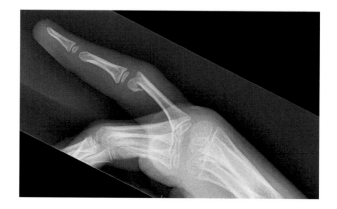

FIGURE 5.15 Off-ended P1 neck fracture in child. This was managed operatively and was irreducible closed so required open reduction and K-wire stabilisation.

deformity they can generally be managed conservatively. If significantly displaced they will require operative management by a senior hand surgeon as they are very difficult to reduce closed (Figure 5.15).

Head Fractures

Phalangeal head fractures (involving the articular surface) are relatively rare and are classified as: (1) Stable fractures without displacement, (2) Unicondylar, unstable fractures, (3) Bicondylar, comminuted unstable fractures. Types 2 and 3 require surgical fixation which is usually with fine percutaneous K-wires [q].

Fractures of Distal Phalanx

Tuft Fractures

Tuft fractures are often associated with nailbed injuries as both are caused by crush injuries (Figure 5.16). The middle

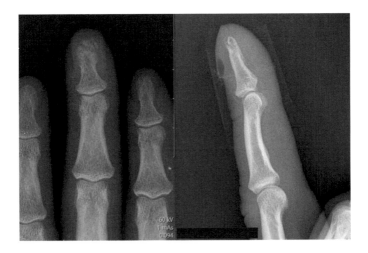

FIGURE 5.16   Tuft fracture of distal phalanx.

finger is most commonly injured followed by the thumb. Tuft fractures, even if comminuted, rarely benefit from surgical intervention. Left to heal, conservatively they may not unite but they clinically heal with fibrous union and there is rarely any long-term functional deficit. As previously mentioned, in the context of an open injury involving the nailbed they can often be reduced by adequate washout and manipulation as part of the process of repairing the nailbed.

Shaft Fractures

Shaft fractures are not only commonly transverse but can also be longitudinal. If they are non-displaced or minimally displaced, they can be immobilised with a zimmer splint and followed up in 1 week with a check X-ray to ensure adequate position has been maintained. If a transverse

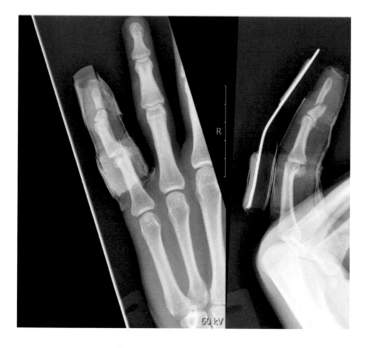

FIGURE 5.17   Displaced transverse midshaft fracture of distal phalanx. This was not improved by manipulation and splinting so required K-wire stabilisation.

(or longitudinal) fracture is significantly displaced then book the patient for MUA and K-wire fixation under LA, as these fractures are generally not amenable to satisfactory reduction with a simple MUA in clinic (Figure 5.17).

For fractures involving the articular surface of P3 see the section on MALLET FINGER.

Dislocations

Dislocations of the MCP and PIP joints are more common than dislocations of the DIP joint. They generally occur due

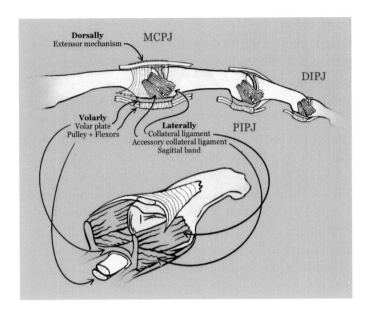

FIGURE 5.18   Box joint complex of finger.

to falls. Dislocations are described according to the position of the distal bone relative to the proximal bone. Every joint can be thought of as a 'box' with stabilising structures on all four sides (Figure 5.18). For the joint to have become dislocated at least two sides of the box has to be disrupted.

An acutely dislocated joint should be relocated as soon as possible to allow assessment of damage to ligamentous structures + treatment (conservative immobilisation or surgical repair). Any dislocation that is more than 1 week old at time of presentation is very hard to reduce closed as in this timeframe the ligaments and tendons associated with the joint will have shortened. This patient group generally requires open surgical reduction ± K-wire stabilisation.

Acute Dislocation

After taking a history and obtaining three-view X-rays of the affected joint including the joint above and below, relocation can be attempted under LA and/or Entonox. Apply firm traction to the affected digit for 2 minutes to bring it out to length. You will need counter traction either from the patient or from a colleague holding their arm. This may be enough to relocate the joint. If you do not feel it pop back then start to apply pressure at the point of the dislocation while maintaining firm traction. If it is the MCPJ that is dislocated then try flexing the wrist as this may aid the relocation. If it is the PIPJ that is affected and will not reduce, it normally means that the volar plate is interposed (stuck) in the joint, which makes non-operative relocation almost impossible. If the dislocation cannot be reduced closed it will require formal reduction in theatre.

If reduction is successful, then assess the following:

- *Active stability:* Ask the patient to move it as far as they are able. Full/nearly full range of movement without spontaneous dislocation indicates that it is stable. If it dislocates on movement, it is unstable.

- *Passive stability:* Assess the integrity of the collateral ligaments at full extension and then at 30 degrees of flexion. For a true comparison compare to an uninjured finger. If there is gross laxity (as indicated by no clear end point) then the patient will require a longer period of immobilisation or may benefit from operative repair of the ligaments. Assess volar and dorsal stability with gentle pressure.

- Obtain new X-rays of the joint to confirm its current position.

If the joint is now relatively stable and there is no gross ligamentous damage then zimmer splint the finger as below for between 1 and 3 weeks depending on severity of injury and refer the patient to hand therapy for follow-up. Request therapy as urgent (within 72 hours).

- Relocated MCP joint = splint in 50 degrees of flexion
- Relocated PIP joint = splint in 20 degrees of flexion
- Relocated DIP joint = splint in slight flexion

Volar Plate Injuries
Volar plate injuries occur from forced hyperextension of a digit. They are most common at the PIPJ. Patients generally present with pain and bruising over the area of the volar plate. Sometimes there is an associated avulsion fracture visible on the lateral view where a small fragment of bone has avulsed with the volar plate. If there is no fracture OR if there is a small, minimally displaced fragment not involving the articular surface, apply a dorsal blocking splint immobilising the affected joint in 20 degrees of flexion and refer the patient to hand therapy for follow up.

If there is a large bone fragment or the fragment is significantly displaced seek senior input as the patient may benefit from a surgical intervention.

Ulnar Collateral Ligament of Thumb
Ulnar collateral ligament (UCL) injuries of the MCP joint of the thumb can occur in the context of a dislocation or as an

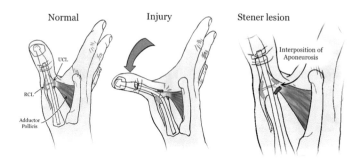

FIGURE 5.19   Anatomy of Stener lesion.

isolated injury. Known as 'Skier's thumb' or 'Gamekeeper's thumb' the injury occurs from forced radial deviation of the thumb. If the UCL is completely ruptured then the patient is very likely to develop a Stener lesion, which is the spontaneous interposition of the adductor pollicis aponeurosis between the ruptured UCL stump and its insertion, meaning that the UCL will not heal with conservative management (Figure 5.19).

Assess the patient as previously described. If there is no end point on clinical assessment of the UCL then book the patient for an exploration ± Mitek bone anchor repair of the UCL. If there is uncertainty about the diagnosis, a USS or (as a gold standard) an MRI can aid the diagnosis. If the UCL rupture is thought to be partial the patient requires 4 weeks of cast immobilisation followed by splint immobilisation and input from the hand therapy team.

CHAPTER 6

Hand and Upper Limb Emergencies

AMPUTATION/REPLANTATION

Significant amputation of digit(s) or the upper limb (Figures 6.1 and 6.2) requires immediate senior input so if you receive a call about an amputation ask the following:

- **What level is the amputation?**

- **Exactly what time did it occur?**

- **What was the mechanism of injury?**

- **How has the amputated part been stored?** If the patient is due to be transferred ask for the amputated part to be wrapped in damp gauze, placed in a zip-lock bag and put on ice (note: it is important that the

DOI: 10.1201/9781003163770-6

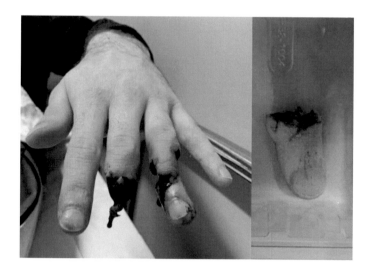

FIGURE 6.1   Presentation + amputate.

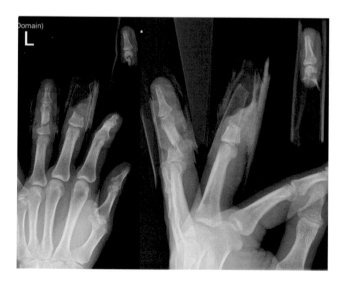

FIGURE 6.2   X-ray of amputation including amputate.

part be prevented from direct contact with the ice, i.e. MUST be wrapped in gauze).

- **Are there any other injuries?**

- **Is the patient stable?**

- **Please send X-rays if they have been carried out.** If not done don't delay transfer to do them.

- **What is the patient's age, occupation, medical background and smoking status?**

Once you have the above information, contact your registrar so they can review the patient with you at the earliest opportunity to decide whether replantation is indicated.

On examination, confirm the level of injury and (with the patient's permission) obtain photographs of the amputated part and stump. Wash the stump with saline only to remove any gross contamination then redress and elevate the limb. Avoid repeatedly manipulating the extremity as this may increase vasospasm and don't do an LA block as this may decrease vascular flow. Obtain three view (AP/Oblique/ Lateral) X-rays of the stump **and** amputated part to aid in surgical planning. Administer tetanus, IV antibiotics, IV fluids, analgesia and make the patient NBM. They will require marking and consenting by the on-call registrar including the following risks (in addition to the normal hand surgery risks):

- Failure of replantation

- Need for bone, nerve, vein graft

- Need for further procedure

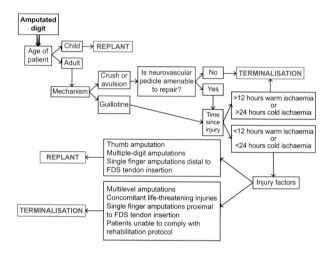

FIGURE 6.3   Indications and contraindications for digit replantation flowchart [r].

Contact the on-call anaesthetist to review the patient, alert the theatre coordinator and book the patient on the emergency board. It is important to do this ASAP as they may need to arrange an additional scrub team for the procedure. Ideally arrange for the patient to be catheterised so their fluid balance can be monitored and because replantation is often a long procedure. Indications and contraindications for digit replantation are as per the above flowchart though every individual case should be discussed with your registrar (Figure 6.3) [r].

In higher level amputations through the hand or forearm replantation is always attempted unless there are significant contraindications such as multi-level amputation, severe crush, significant other injuries or severe medical co-morbidities.

KEY MANAGEMENT POINTS

- Amputation is a surgical emergency – involve your senior immediately.
- Ensure initial management steps completed including correct management of amputated part, IV antibiotics, tetanus, X-rays of hand and amputate, history of time and mechanism of the injury.

COMPARTMENT SYNDROME OF UPPER LIMB

Compartment syndrome is a limb-threatening condition in which increased pressure within a closed (fascial) compartment compromises blood flow to muscles and nerves. If untreated it leads rapidly to tissue ischaemia and necrosis, which can ultimately result in loss of function, loss of limb, rhabdomyolysis and renal compromise. In the upper limb, compartment syndrome most commonly affects the deep compartment of the forearm but it can also affect other compartments of the forearm, hand and (less commonly) the upper arm. Acute compartment syndrome is a surgical emergency for which the only definitive management is decompression with fasciotomies. Time to theatres is crucial as irreversible tissue injury starts at approximately 3 hours of warm ischemia with 6 hours as the upper limit of muscle viability.

Compartment syndrome is caused by either an increase of volume within the compartment (swelling) or a decrease of volume imposed on the compartment (compression) (Table 6.1).

TABLE 6.1   Causes of Compartment Syndrome

Increased Volume (Swelling)	Decreased Volume (Compression)
Fractures/dislocations (most common cause)	Overly tight dressing/cast
Crush injury	Circumferential full thickness burns
Haemorrhage	Prolonged limb positioning during surgery
Ischaemia reperfusion injury	
Oedema due to electrical burn	
Strenuous muscle use	

Following an insult, the pressure within a compartment slowly rises, and if it reaches approximately 30 mmHg of intra-compartmental pressure the venous capillaries collapse, leading to a decrease in venous outflow. Due to arterial pressure being higher than 30 mmHg, the arterial inflow to the compartment continues, so the intra-compartmental pressure then rapidly rises in a vicious cycle that leads to full blown compartment syndrome.

Have a high index of suspicion for potential compartment syndrome in any patient with one of the above listed injuries/insults. In particular, keep compartment syndrome in mind in any patient with a long bone injury, a high velocity injury, a crush or stabbing injury.

It is a clinical diagnosis. On reviewing the patient, the main sign of evolving compartment syndrome is *pain out of proportion to the injury*, often not responding in the normal way to analgesia. On examination, the most sensitive test is pain on palpation and on passive stretch of the compartment. Paraesthesia indicates early nerve ischaemia. The other well-known indicators of compartment syndrome are late signs, which make them unhelpful diagnostically (pulselessness, paralysis, pallor, poikilothermia or 'perishingly cold'). In an alert patient, convincing clinical findings in the context of an appropriate insult is enough to make the diagnosis of compartment syndrome and to prompt an emergency fasciotomy.

Fasciotomy of the forearm requires one volar incision to decompress the superficial and deep compartments and one dorsal incision to decompress the dorsal compartment. Fasciotomy of the hand requires decompression of the carpal tunnel, thenar and hypothenar eminences and two dorsal incisions to decompress the deep compartments of the hand (five incisions in total). Fasciotomy of the upper arm requires a medial and lateral fasciotomy. Warn the patient about scarring and the need for later skin grafts (Figure 6.4).

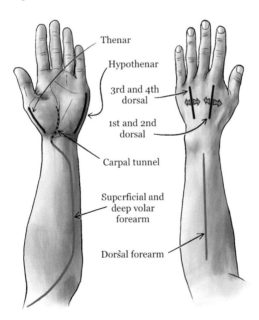

FIGURE 6.4   Fasciotomy incisions of forearm and hand.

HIGH PRESSURE INJECTION

High-pressure injection injuries to the hand or forearm are a surgical emergency that require urgent exploration and debridement to avoid severe inflammation, infection and potential loss of the affected limb/digit (Figures 6.5, 6.6 and 6.7).

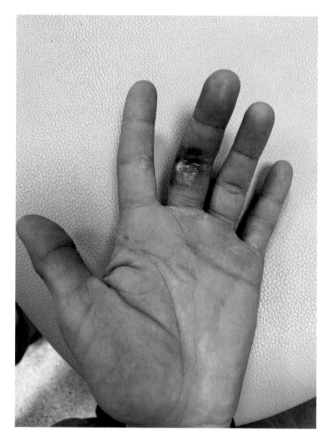

FIGURE 6.5   Note white paint visible + swelling of finger. Yellow is from inadine dressing.

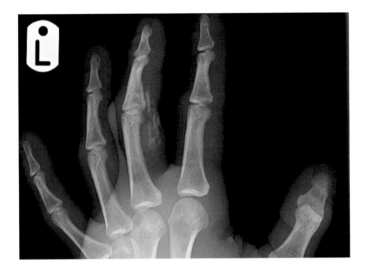

FIGURE 6.6   Paint visible on X-ray.

They are generally sustained to the non-dominant hand when using a commercial paint spray gun. By definition the entry point will be small and may appear unimpressive but without urgent surgical debridement the tissue that has been infiltrated by the aerosol will become compromised over 24–48 hours due to a combination of inflammation ± compartment syndrome ± infection.

Take a history including the time of injury, what was injected and any first aid to date. Order X-rays as they may show the extent of the infiltration of the chemical and admit for same day emergency washout. Wash, dress, splint and elevate the affected hand. Prescribe analgesia, IV antibiotics, tetanus and make the patient nil by mouth. Monitor the affected limb for worsening pain suggestive of impending compartment syndrome.

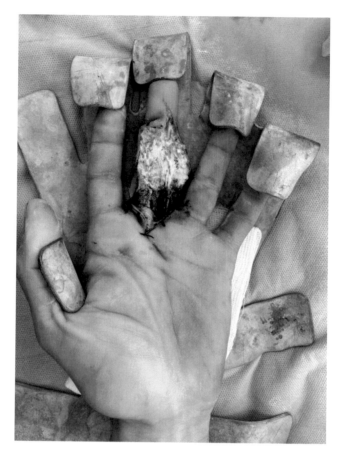

FIGURE 6.7   White paint widespread in deep tissues of finger.

KEY MANAGEMENT POINT

- High pressure injection is a surgical emergency requiring admission and same-day washout.

FINGER DEGLOVING

Degloving of the finger is a relatively rare but often severe injury sustained by avulsion of a ring worn by the patient. Commonly the ring is caught in machinery in a workplace accident or caught as the patient descends a fence. Classification and general approach to management is as per below table.

Degloving Type	Description	Management
I	Soft tissue injury *without* vascular compromise.	Admit and consent for emergency (but not immediate) surgical exploration and reconstruction. N.B. depending on extent of tissue loss these patients may require a local flap or skin graft.
II	Soft tissue injury *with* vascular compromise.	Admit and **seek immediate senior input** as may be amenable to revascularisation to salvage the finger.
III	Complete degloving of soft tissues (skeletalisation).	Admit and consent for primary ray amputation.

If you receive a referral about a ring avulsion, ask the following:

- **Exactly what time did it occur?**
- **What was the mechanism of injury?**

- **Are there any other injuries?**

- **Is the tip of the finger perfused?**

- **Is the patient stable?**

- **Please send X-rays if they have been carried out.** (If not done don't delay transfer to do them.)

- **What is the patient's age, occupation, medical background and smoking status?**

Once you have the above information contact your registrar so they can review the patient with you at the earliest opportunity.

On examination, assess perfusion by checking warmth and capillary refill time at the tip. Examine the wound to ascertain whether it is likely that both neurovascular bundles have been compromised. Avoid using a ring block as this can decrease vascular flow.

Hand dominance, occupation, co-morbidities and smoking status are important parts of the history in this patient group especially if there is a type II injury that may or may not survive a revascularisation attempt. For instance, a self-employed manual worker (keen to return to work) who is also a smoker (poor wound healing) may elect for amputation over a revascularisation attempt.

KEY MANAGEMENT POINTS
- Admit + IV antibiotics + tetanus + elevate + NBM.
- Seek senior input immediately.

EXTRAVASATION

Extravasation is the leaking of fluid or medication into extra vascular tissue from an intravenous device. Most commonly it is small to moderate volumes of saline or IV contrast that have been extravasated, which rarely have severe consequences, but depending on the fluid type and the volume extravasated there are the potential serious complications of full thickness skin loss and compartment syndrome. For this reason, any extravasation referrals must be urgently investigated with the following questions:

- **What substance has been extravasated?**
- **What volume has been extravasated?**
- **Exactly what time did it occur?**
- **Any initial management?**
- **General clinical condition of patient?**

Ask the referring clinician to aspirate from the cannula as this may remove some of the extravasated fluid. Make it clear that the cannula should not be used and should not be flushed. Ask them to leave the cannula in and elevate the limb immediately in a Bradford sling or on pillows. Attend the patient as soon as you are able and with particular urgency if involvement of a vesicant (blister producing chemical) OR paediatric patient OR large volume of fluid.

On attending the patient examine the area of extravasation and the limb distal to the site. If the cannula is still in you can attempt a further aspiration with gentle pressure on the affected area, then remove the cannula. Document skin appearance including colour and blistering and if there are skin changes mark the border of the affected skin. Examine the limb distal to the extravasation assessing swelling and compartment tenderness. Check CRT, sensation, movement, pulses and clearly document all findings.

If the skin appears uncompromised and you have no acute concerns about compartment syndrome ensure the limb is elevated and make a plan to review it again – ideally within an hour or two. Extravasation injuries can continue to evolve for up to 5 days. If there is severe blistering OR signs of skin necrosis OR concern of compartment syndrome OR the substance extravasated is a vesicant involve your senior immediately to review the patient with you.

Saline or hylase washout should be considered for extravasation with high-risk vesicants such as chemotherapy agents. Check local policy on this when starting at the unit. Anaesthetise the skin around the extravasation site with LA and make some stab incisions through the skin. Slowly inject 0.9% sterile saline from the peripheries of the affected area into the affected area to flush the soft tissues (Figure 6.8). Having passed through the soft tissues, fluid exits through the incisions [s]. As a rule of thumb use a total volume of saline that is at least twice the volume of the vesicant that was extravasated. Then cold compress, elevation and further review.

In cases of severe soft tissue damage, local antidote infiltration may be beneficial (Table 6.2). Corticosteroids or hyaluronidase can be used for chemotherapy agents (https://extravasation.org.uk/CEG.htm), phentolamine for vasopressors and hyaluronidase for hyperosmolar agents [t]. Seek senior input before initiating this treatment.

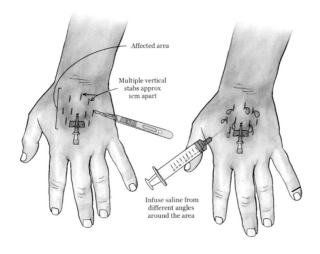

FIGURE 6.8   Saline washout of extravasation site.

TABLE 6.2   Extravasation Fluids + Antidotes

Hyperosmolar Solutions	Non-physiological pH	Vasopressors	Cytotoxic Drugs
Fluids	*Acidic*	Adrenaline	Actinomycin
		Noradrenaline	Amrubicin
10–50% glucose	Amiodarone	Dopamine	Amsacrine
3% saline	Amphotericin	Dobutamine	Azathiaprine
Parenteral	Caffeine	Vasopressin	Carmustine
nutrition	Cefotaxime	Phenylephrine	Dacarbazine
(TPN)	Co-trimoxazole	Prostaglandins	Dactinomycin
Potassium	Doxycycline		Daunorubicin
chloride	Gentamicin	*Antidote:*	Docetaxel
>40 mmol/L		Phentolamine	Doxorubicin
Mannitol			Epirubicin
			Idarubicin
Medications	Metronidazole		Mitomycin
	Pentamidine		

(Continued)

TABLE 6.2   Extravasation Fluids + Antidotes *(Continued)*

Hyperosmolar Solutions	Non-physiological pH	Vasopressors	Cytotoxic Drugs
Calcium solutions	Promethazine		Mustine
Diazepam	Vancomycin		Paclitexel
Digoxin			Streptozocin
Lorazepam			Treosulfan
Magnesium sulphate 20 or 50%	*Alkali*		Vinblastine
			Vincristine
Nitroglycerin			
Phenobarbitone			
Phenytoin	Aciclovir		
	Ampicillin		
Potassium phosphate	Aminophylline		
	Erythromycin		
Radiographic contrast	Foscarnet sodium		
	Ganciclovir		
Sodium bicarbonate	Phenytoin		
	Thiopentone		**ANTIDOTE: Corticosteroids ± hyaluronidase**
ANTIDOTE: Hyaluronidase			

KEY MANAGEMENT POINTS

- Gather information on timing + fluid type + fluid amount when taking extravasation referral.
- Urgently attend extravasation, as if washout is required the sooner the better.
- Elevate and monitor for 48 hours.

CHAPTER 7

Necrotising Fasciitis

Necrotising fasciitis (NF) is a life-threatening surgical emergency. It is a rapidly progressing soft tissue infection that can only be controlled by immediate debridement in theatres to save the patient's limb/life (Figures 7.1 and 7.2).

Pathophysiology: In NF bacteria release toxins that cause inflammation and necrosis of surrounding tissue. It spreads rapidly along fascial planes but does not infiltrate into muscle.

Risk factors: Diabetes, obesity, immunosuppression, IV drug use, advanced age and haematological malignancy increase the risk of NF. However, it can also occur in young and healthy patients.

Microbiology: NF is split into three main types according to causative organisms.

DOI: 10.1201/9781003163770-7   **111**

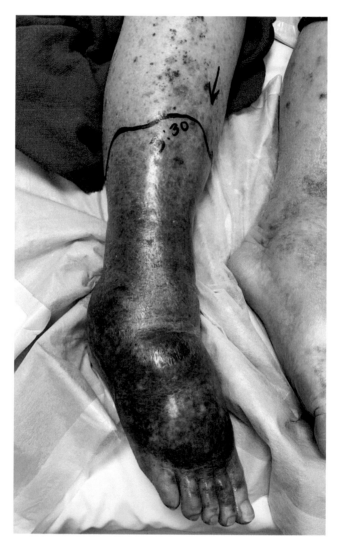

FIGURE 7.1 Acute late presentation of necrotising fasciitis of leg.

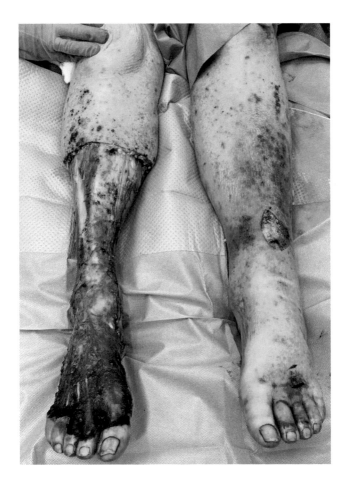

FIGURE 7.2   Same patient post-initial debridement.

Gas gangrene is rarer than types 1 and 2; however, it progresses more rapidly and is often fatal as toxins produced by the *Clostridium* organisms can necrose muscle and cause myocardial depression (Table 7.1). Definitive diagnosis of the infective organism (through cultures) takes time

TABLE 7.1   Necrotising Fasciitis Types

Type 1	Polymicrobial	Most common overall. Often involves Group A *Streptococcus.* Other common organisms include *Bacteroides, Clostridium, Pseudomonas, E. coli, Klebsiella, Peptostreptococcus* and *Proteus* [v]
Type 2	Monomicrobial	Generally Group A *Streptococcus*
Type 3	Gas gangrene/clostridial myonecrosis	Generally *Clostridium perfringens.* Also other types of clostridium bacteria such as alpha toxin or theta toxin

and makes no difference in the emergency management of this condition.

Aetiology: NF usually follows a traumatic wound, which may be as small as an insect bite or scratch. NF may also develop from sites of intravenous drug injection or sites of 'contaminated' surgery such as bowel surgery or gynaecological surgery. Fournier's gangrene is necrotising fasciitis of the scrotum. This condition can be precipitated by trauma, surgery, scrotal abscess, urinary tract infection and ureteric stones.

Presentation: Initially flu-like symptoms such as nausea, fever, diarrhoea, dizziness and general malaise. There may be pain at and around the infection site which can be severe BUT pain may be absent in patients with neuropathy. As the infection progresses, patients commonly display high fever and clinical signs of sepsis including tachycardia and hypotension. Severe, constant pain at the infection point that is out of proportion to the original injury is characteristic of NF. Swelling and a progressing red/purple rash at the site of the infection is common. The rash darkens and blisters form. Skin necrosis then starts with blackening of the skin. If left unmanaged, decreased sensation in the affected area occurs due to death of sensory nerves. Spontaneous splitting of the skin releasing grey, foul smelling fluid is a late sign.

Diagnosis: Early diagnosis is difficult. Have a high index of suspicion in any unwell patient with significant soft tissue infection, particularly if they have the aforementioned medical risk factors AND/OR are not responding to antibiotic treatment. Surgical exploration is the only way to accurately confirm or exclude NF.

The affected area may demonstrate crepitus on palpation which is caused by air. In this instance, the likely diagnosis is of gas gangrene caused by bacteria of the clostridium group. This distinction makes no difference to acute management which remains emergency surgical debridement.

The 'finger test' is a bedside test where a 2–3 cm incision is made over the affected area after infiltration with local anaesthetic. Leakage of dishwater-grey coloured fluid is indicative of NF, as is absence of bleeding. The ability to gently sweep a surgically gloved finger through the fascial layer with minimal resistance is again indicative of NF. Check with your registrar if they want to perform this test as in many cases it is bypassed in the diagnosis of NF.

TABLE 7.2   Laboratory Risk Indicator Score for Necrotizing Fasciitis (LRINEC)

Marker	Value	LRINEC Score
C-reactive protein, mg/L	<150	0
	≥150	4
Total white cell count, per mm^3	<15	0
	15–25	1
	>25	2
Haemoglobin, g/L	>135	0
	110–135	1
	<110	2
Sodium, mmol/L	≥135	0
	<135	2
Creatinine, μmol/L	≤141	0
	>141	2
Glucose, mmol/L	≤10	0
	>10	1

The laboratory risk indicator score for necrotising fasciitis (LRINEC) score may be helpful when assessing a patient although there is limited evidence for its efficacy (Table 7.2) [w]. Patients scoring greater than 6 should be evaluated carefully for NF.

A total LRINEC score of ≥6 is a reasonable cut-off to rule *in* necrotizing fasciitis but **a score of <6 does not exclude the diagnosis**.

The benefit of imaging versus the delay in treatment means that it is generally not used in the diagnosis of NF. Subcutaneous emphysema may be seen on X-ray. CT and MRI can aid diagnosis of early NF but can create an unacceptable delay in treatment [x].

When you receive a referral querying necrotising fasci-itis, it is therefore important to get a full medical picture of the patient including:

- Underlying risk factors

- Clinical progression since admission

- Current clinical status including:

  - Observations

  - Recent blood tests (if not available ask for them to be done immediately)

  - Recent and current anti-microbial therapy

  - Recent ABG/VBG (if not available ask for one to be done immediately)

- Surgical and anaesthetic history including when last ate

Ask for the patient to be made nil by mouth and IV fluids to be started pending assessment. Early administration of empirical broad-spectrum IV antibiotics according to local protocols is essential (typically including clindamycin in addition to a high dose penicillin and aminoglycoside). If the description is of a septic patient ask for the referring team to involve critical care. Attend urgently.

Management: As previously stated NF is a surgical emergency which requires immediate debridement in theatres. Initial debridement should be carried out *at the patient's current hospital* by an available surgeon (general, urology, orthopaedics or plastics are all able to do the initial debridement). Under no circumstances should a patient with presumed NF who is potentially unstable be transferred to another hospital for plastic surgery input in the emergency setting. Once stabilised, patients can be transferred to a plastic surgery unit for reconstruction.

Debridement is carried out down to viable tissue and depending on the progression of the infection may be radical. Patients require at least two serial debridements with sending of tissue samples to ensure full control and clearance of infected tissue before any reconstruction can be planned. Local antibiotic guidelines should be followed and microbiology advice should be sought.

KEY MANAGEMENT POINTS

- Necrotising fasciitis is a life-threatening surgical emergency.
- Though lab tests and imaging can serve as useful adjuncts the diagnosis is a clinical diagnosis. As such if there is suspicion of NF then involve your senior immediately.
- While you await their review prepare the patient for theatres – NBM, consent and book, IV fluids, IV antibiotics as per trust protocol, bloods including group and save.

CHAPTER **8**

Lower Limb Trauma

Referrals to plastics for lower limb trauma are always regarding soft tissue coverage.

At one end of the injury severity spectrum are pretibial lacerations, which often only require a clinical review and dressings advice. At the other end of the spectrum are high energy open fractures or degloving injuries of the leg, which require complex flap reconstruction working closely with the Trauma and Orthopaedics (T&O) team.

PRETIBIAL LACERATIONS AND HAEMATOMAS

Low energy injuries to the shin can lead to skin tears or flaps known as pretibial lacerations (Figure 8.1). These injuries are most common in elderly patients and often result from blunt trauma such as a fall, or a simple knock against furniture. The skin in this region has poor collagen integrity, especially in the elderly and patients on steroid treatment, which means that it is fragile. In the

DOI: 10.1201/9781003163770-8

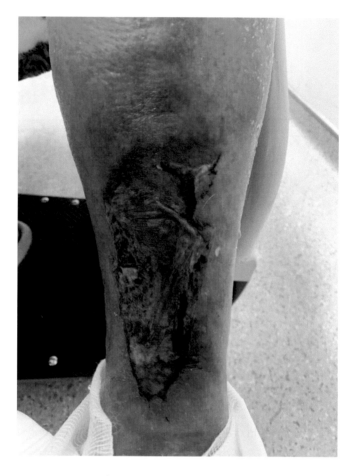

FIGURE 8.1 Dunkin grade II pretibial laceration. Though the affected area is approximately 1% TBSA, the devitalisation of the skin was not full thickness. This patient was therefore treated by washing the wound + trimming the necrotic superficial skin flap, then with serial dressings and wound monitoring. If the wound had been deeper, they would have required a split thickness skin graft.

anti-coagulated patient, these injuries can also result in rupture of perforators and subsequent haematoma formation. Pressure caused by an expanding haematoma can compromise the overlying skin leading to skin necrosis and skin loss.

If seen acutely, washing and approximating the skin edges ± evacuation of any haematoma is the optimal management for most pretibial lacerations. However, if there is a significant amount of skin loss or degloving (>1% TBSA) or if there is skin necrosis due to a haematoma then a formal procedure to debride and cover the defect with a split thickness skin graft is required (Figure 8.2).

As an SHO you need to initially manage the injury, and to organise appropriate follow-up. If operative management is required it may be as an emergency day case or

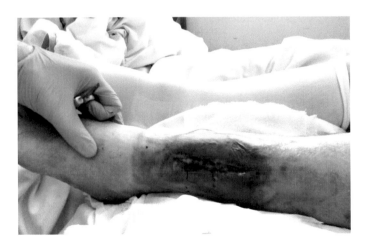

FIGURE 8.2   Dunkin grade III pretibial haematoma. Drainage of this haematoma in ED was unsuccessful (due to delay in presentation) so formal surgical debridement + SSG was required.

the patient may need admitting – check with your registrar. If the patient does need to be admitted check their co-morbidities as it may be wise to have them under joint care with the medical team.

History

When receiving referrals for a pretibial injury check the following:

- What was the mechanism of injury?
  - Low energy or high energy + clues about potential contamination.
  - If was not a mechanical fall: Does this patient require a medical review?
  - Has a secondary survey been completed?
- Exactly when did the injury happen? (Delayed presentation more likely have compromised skin viability, desiccation and infection)
- Has an open fracture has been ruled out?
- Is the limb swollen? (Expanding haematoma should be considered.)

On reviewing the patient check the following:

- Full PMH with a focus on vascular status. (This will help guide management options as they influence wound healing. Diabetes, peripheral vascular disease, peripheral oedema and smoking status should be considered.)

- Drug history (Specifically check for steroids, antiplatelets and anticoagulants – consider switching patient to bridging therapy if they require a procedure.)

- Falls history, mobility status and social history (This will be required to ensure a safe discharge with adequate package of care.)

Examination and Management

Management is guided by Dunkin Classification of pretibial injuries grades from I to IV, with management recommendations [aa] (Table 8.1).

Prior to examination, ensure that pain is adequately managed. This could include local anaesthetic, oral analgesia, and Entonox.

For Dunkin grade I or II pretibial lacerations, wash the wound with sterile saline and aim for tension free approximation of the skin edges. Broad Steristrips are useful for achieving this. Then dress with a non-adherent interface (e.g. Mepitel), gauze and a gentle pressure bandage (wool and crepe). Reduction of oedema is important in increasing dermal perfusion; however, pressure dressings need to be used with caution as they can result in tissue necrosis if applied too tightly. Advise the patient to elevate the leg when at rest but to continue to mobilise normally [bb]. Advise them to keep the dressing dry and book a district nurse or plastics dressings clinic wound review within 7 days. All being well this patient group will not require further plastics follow up and will be managed with serial dressing changes.

There is insufficient evidence for prophylactic use of antibiotics in pretibial lacerations; however, if there is

TABLE 8.1   Dunkin Classification of Pretibial Injuries and
Management Recommendations [aa]

Dunkin Grade	Description	Management Recommendation
	Laceration	Clean with saline SteriStrip™ without tension Apply Supportive dressing
	Laceration or flap with minimal haematoma and/or skin edge necrosis	Clean with saline Trim non-viable skin/tissue Evacuate haematoma SteriStrip™ without tension Apply Supportive dressing
	Laceration or flap with moderate to severe haematoma and/or necrosis	Trim non-viable skin/tissue Split-skin graft under anaesthesia (generally under LA)
	Major degloving injury	Debride non-viable tissue Reconstruct under general anaesthesia

contamination or any signs of infection have a low threshold to give antibiotics as these wounds are prone to infection [bb].

Small-to moderate-sized **acute** pretibial haematomas in a stable patient can generally be evacuated in the emergency department under LA/Entonox. Prepare adequate dressings including a non-adherent interface, lots of gauze, wool and crepe to create a pressure dressing. Make a small incision (3–4 cm) in the skin over the haematoma and squeeze out the blood. Wash the wound. Be aware that the haematoma is likely to reaccumulate without an adequate pressure dressing (particularly if the patient is on anticoagulants) so quickly apply your dressings, elevate the leg and observe for a few minutes to check that bleeding is controlled. Advise the patient to strictly keep the dressing dry. Depending on the size of the haematoma and condition of the skin you may want to arrange a formal wound review within 2–3 days, or alternatively nurse led review within 1 week.

If the haematoma is **over a day old** the blood may be difficult to evacuate due to coagulation. In this instance the decision as to whether to evacuate it is made on a case-by-case basis depending on the viability of the overlying skin and age of the haematoma – consult your senior.

For Dunkin III or IV pretibial haematomas (i.e. which involve a large full thickness necrotic skin flap OR an area of full thickness skin loss greater than 1% TBSA OR a major haematoma) liaise with your registrar regarding management. Wash and dress the wound. Depending on the severity of the injury, co-morbidities of the patient and available operating lists it will become clear whether it is better to admit the patient or to plan an emergency day case procedure. Request pre-op bloods including clotting screen and consult a haematologist regarding bridging therapy if the patient is on anticoagulants/antiplatelets.

OPEN FRACTURES OF THE LOWER LIMB

Lower limb open fractures are severe injuries, which exposure bone and deep tissues to the outer environment. In order to avoid infection with the potential sequelae of amputation or sepsis these injuries require prompt management as per the BOAST guidelines (British Orthopaedic Association Standards for Trauma and Orthopaedics) [cc].

Lower limb open fractures are sustained by two patient groups (broadly speaking). The first of these are young male patients with high energy injuries from road traffic accidents and interpersonal violence. The second group is elderly patients with low energy injuries from falls [dd].

The role of plastics in management of these injuries is in planning soft tissue coverage which could be anything from direct closure, a local flap or a free flap (Figures 8.3 and 8.4). Referral to plastics for these injuries is commonly made after completion of primary and secondary surveys by the Trauma and Orthopaedic team (T&O). Your role as an SHO is to gather information on the injury including (with the patient's permission) images of the injury. This information will enable your senior to start formulating a plan for soft tissue coverage. Ultimately, the decision as to how to manage the wound is made by a consultant plastic surgeon in discussion with a consultant orthopaedic surgeon in theatres at the time of initial debridement.

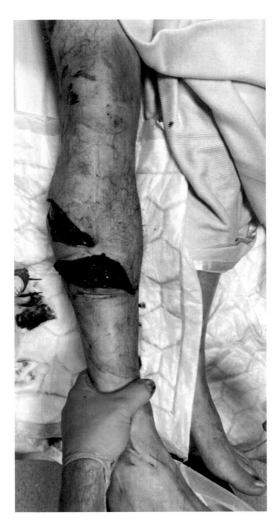

FIGURE 8.3   Open fracture of tibia post-reduction. On debridement this was found to be a Gustilo IIIB, i.e. inadequate soft tissue coverage of fracture site. After fracture fixation the defect was reconstructed with a free flap.

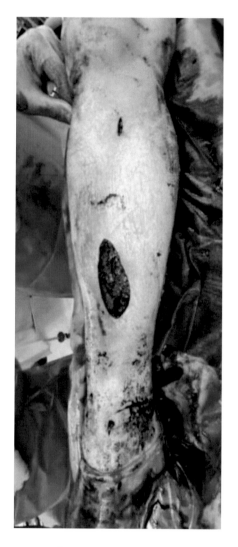

FIGURE 8.4   Open fracture of tibia. On debridement this was found to be a Gustilo IIIA, i.e. high energy injury with defect just over 10 cm but adequate soft tissue coverage available.

History

On receiving a referral for an open lower limb fracture find out the following:

- Patient age
- Time and mechanism of injury
- If polytrauma + details of other injuries
- Current resuscitation status
- Current neurovascular status of the limb
- Details of the fracture
- Current orthopaedic plan
- Results of any investigations (bloods/imaging/ vascular studies)
- Past medical history + medications + allergies
- Time since last ate & drank

Alert your registrar about the referral and attend the patient in ED.

Examination

Ensure that the patient has been assessed and stabilised as per ATLS principles. Before you can examine the wound the T&O team need to have realigned the fracture – check this has taken place. Key parts of your examination are as follows:

1. **Wound assessment + initial wound management**

   - Expose and photograph the wound. Include joints above and below in the photos so anatomy is clear, e.g. for open tibia/fibula fracture include the ankle and knee.

- Document the following: Size, location, shape of wound and if contaminated as well as if actively bleeding.

- If the wound is clean, it should not be handled or washed – simply dress with a saline soaked gauze and cover with an occlusive dressing.

- If there is gross contamination the wound is handled only to remove the contamination. Thereafter simply dress with saline soaked gauze and an occlusive dressing.

2. **Vascularity of limb distal to injury**

- Foot colour (? pale) & temperature (? cool)

- Capillary refill time

- Palpate dorsalis pedis and posterior tibial pulses (? strong/weak. Mark with a pen where you felt them.)

- If pulses not palpable assess with Doppler.

- If you have any concerns that vascularity is compromised alert your senior immediately + book urgent CT angiogram.

3. **Nerves**

- Common peroneal nerve: This is susceptible to injury in fibular head fractures. To test motor function, ask the patient to dorsiflex the foot. To test sensation check in 1st webspace of dorsum of foot (deep peroneal branch).

- Tibial nerve: To test motor check plantar flexion of foot.

Clearly and fully document your examination to demonstrate, you have checked these important elements (and in case of any future deterioration of the patient).

Management

Initial BOAST management is often carried out by the T&O team but for safety, ensure the following steps have been completed:

- Prophylactic IV antibiotics as per trust protocol have been given within 1 hour of the injury (BOAST guideline).

- Tetanus shot given/up to date with tetanus (BOAST guideline).

- Prophylactic dose low-molecular-weight heparin prescribed.

- Secondary survey completed.

- Appropriate analgesia and fluid resuscitation of patient given.

- Two orthogonal view X-rays of fracture site including joint above and below.

Additional key points:

- If fracture site is manipulated or splinted then the neurovascular status **must** be re-checked and clearly documented.

- Any patient with a lower limb fracture should be monitored for compartment syndrome of the lower limb.

- The following are absolute indications for immediate formal surgical debridement regardless of time of day. If any of these are present the plastics consultant on call needs to be made aware immediately:

  - Wound highly contaminated (marine, agricultural or sewage).

  - Arterial damage compromising circulation to distal leg.

  - Compartment syndrome compromising circulation to distal leg.

- If none of the above are present then the patient needs to be worked up for debridement and planning of soft tissue coverage on the next available daytime consultant led joint orthoplastics list. As per BOAST 4 guidelines this debridement should take place within 12 hours for solitary high energy open fractures or within 24 hours for low energy open fractures.

Gustilo Anderson Classification

There exist a number of lower limb injury scoring systems but it is the Gustilo Anderson Classification that is most broadly used (Table 8.2). An injury can only formally be

TABLE 8.2 Gustilo Anderson Classification

| Feature | Fracture Type | | | | |
	I	II	IIIA	IIIB	IIIC
Wound size (cm)	<1	1–10	>10	>10	Any size
Energy	Low	Moderate	High	High	High
Contamination	Minimal	Moderate	Severe	Severe	Severe
Deep soft tissue damage	Minimal	Moderate	Severe	Severe	Severe
Fracture comminution	Minimal	Moderate	Severe/segmental	Severe/segmental	Severe/segmental
Periosteal stripping	No	No	Yes	Yes	Yes
Local coverage	Adequate	Adequate	Adequate	**Inadequate**	**Inadequate**
Arterial compromise	No	No	No	No	**Yes**

134 ■ Plastic Surgery for Trauma

given a Gustilo Anderson classification **at the time of debridement in theatres**. However, it is common to hear colleagues describing an injury by Gustilo Anderson classification based on the initial assessment in resus, the reason being that it is a useful way to communicate the (suspected) severity of the injury.

Immediate vascular operative involvement is required for IIIC injuries as circulation is compromised. Plastics operative involvement is required for type IIIB and IIIC injuries as in these injuries there is inadequate soft tissue coverage of the bone (see below in bold).

Compartment Syndrome of the Lower Limb

Compartment syndrome is a limb-threatening surgical emergency in which increased pressure within a closed (fascial) compartment compromises blood flow to muscles and nerves. For information on pathophysiology and aetiology of compartment syndrome see page 121.

In high-energy lower limb trauma, compartment syndrome is common due to the elements of significant soft tissue injury (particularly crush) + fracture. If there is vascular injury then compartment syndrome can also occur as a result of reperfusion post-vessel repair. For this reason, patients with open lower limb fractures need to be *carefully monitored for signs of impending compartment syndrome* [ee]. Of the four compartments in the calf, it is the anterior then the lateral compartments most commonly affected.

Clinical Assessment

Compartment syndrome is a clinical diagnosis. On reviewing the patient, the main sign of evolving compartment syndrome is *pain out of proportion to the injury*, often not responding in the normal way to analgesia. Pain from compartment syndrome gets progressively worse over the course of a few hours so if you see a patient in whom this is occurring – think compartment syndrome.

On examination, the most sensitive test is *severe pain on passive stretch of the compartment*. Passively plantar flex the ankle and great toe to test the anterior and lateral compartments of the lower leg. Passively dorsiflex the ankle and great toe to test the posterior compartments (Figure 8.5).

Check sensation. *Paraesthesia (numbness or tingling) indicates early nerve ischaemia* and may be present. For example,

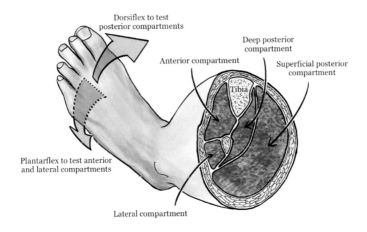

FIGURE 8.5   Lower leg compartments.

altered sensation in the first dorsal webspace of the foot is suggestive of deep peroneal nerve ischaemia secondary to compartment syndrome of the anterior compartment.

The other well-known signs of compartment syndrome are late signs, which makes them unhelpful diagnostically (pulselessness, paralysis, pallor, poikilothermia or 'perishingly cold'). In an alert patient with a lower limb fracture, convincing clinical findings is enough to make the diagnosis of compartment syndrome and to prompt an emergency fasciotomy.

If you suspect compartment syndrome do the following:

1. Release the patient's cast (if any).

2. Immediately inform your senior as the patient may need an emergency fasciotomy.

3. Stop any anticoagulants – check with haematology if bridging required.

4. Send bloods including U&E, creatine kinase (CK) and myoglobin – to monitor potential rhabdomyolysis.

In a patient with a reduced GCS (due to polytrauma ± sedation) and in young children, examination findings are limited, so compartment syndrome can be easily missed. In this patient group the gold standard is to measure intra-compartmental pressure directly with a hand-held manometer (e.g. Stryker manometer – Figure 8.6). A needle is inserted into each compartment to check pressures. If such a device is not available an 18-gauge needle can be attached to an arterial line pressure monitor and inserted into the compartments to measure pressures.

Normal intra-compartmental pressure is <10 mmHg. If the measured pressure is

- Higher than 30 mmHg OR

- Within 30 mmHg of the diastolic blood pressure, i.e. diastolic pressure *minus* intra-compartmental pressure = less than 30 mmHg

This indicates compartment syndrome and the patient requires an emergency fasciotomy. As an SHO you are very unlikely to be asked to carry out this test but it is good to be aware of the process.

If a patient requires a decompression, the role of plastics is to assist the T&O team performing the fasciotomy. The reason for plastics involvement is that there is a risk that a fasciotomy can damage perforator vessels that may later be needed for local flap coverage of the traumatic wound.

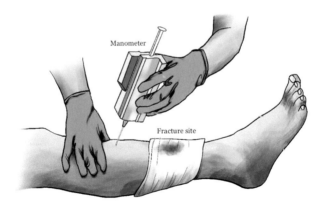

FIGURE 8.6   Checking of anterior compartment pressure with a handheld manometer device.

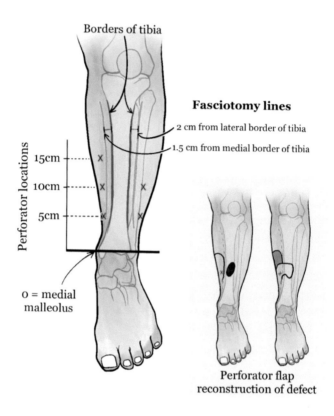

Borders of tibia

Fasciotomy lines

2 cm from lateral border of tibia

1.5 cm from medial border of tibia

Perforator locations

15cm

10cm

5cm

0 = medial malleolus

Perforator flap reconstruction of defect

FIGURE 8.7 Optimal fasciotomy lines to preserve perforators in case they are required for local flap reconstruction.

If (as per the below diagram) the fasciotomy lines are placed 1.5–2 cm on either side of the palpable anterior part of the tibia, then the perforators will lie BEHIND the fasciotomy lines. If a local flap (such as a rotational flap) is later needed for soft tissue reconstruction then the opportunity to raise the flap on one of these perforators remains.

CHAPTER 9

Burns

Burns range from minor injuries requiring advice on dressings and outpatient follow-up to major life-threatening
injuries. Depending on the nature of where you are working
you may be required to assess and manage burns anywhere
along this spectrum.

Within the UK, national guidelines exist on when a
referral should be made to a specialist burns service [ff].
ED staff should know when to make these referrals, and at
the unit receiving the referral (normally a burns centre) the
referrals are routinely triaged by specialist nurses. For this
reason, in most Plastics units *you are unlikely to receive a
direct referral about a major resus burn.* If you DO receive
such a referral, you should ask immediately if a referral has
also been made to the regional burns centre. If the patient
has already arrived at your (non-burns centre) hospital
your role will be to carry out an initial assessment and to
ensure the patient is stabilised before being transferred to

the regional burns centre. You will not be expected to do this alone. Involve your registrar, the ED staff and on call anaesthetist to help in the management of any major or complex burn. Criteria for referral to burns service can be found at the end of the chapter.

RECEIVING BURNS REFERRAL

When you receive a referral about a burn ask the following key questions:

- What time exactly did the burn occur?

- What was the mechanism of the burn? (scald/flame/chemical/electrical)

- If scald: What was the liquid? If chemical: What was the chemical? If electrical: What was the voltage?

- Was the patient inside? If so what sort of space? (Enclosed space increases risk of inhalation injury)

- How long were they exposed to the source of the burn?

- Who else was there at the time? (Ideally get collateral history if possible)

- What first aid was given at the time? How long was it given for? (Longer cool water was run the better)

- What treatment has been given since? (Dressings, analgesia, fluids, tetanus)

- Standard medical history + AMPLE history.

BURNS FIRST AID

Though first aid should have been completed by the time you see a patient in ED a knowledge of the basic principles is required.

Thermal burns:

• Remove clothing and any jewellery in or near-burned area (rings necklaces earrings). Note: If clothing is stuck on do not rip it off.

• Irrigate the burn with cool (but not iced) running water for **20–30 minutes** (note: irrigation can have some affect up to 3 hours post burn).

• Post-irrigation, cover the burn with clingfilm or clean cotton sheet.

• Do not use topical creams.

• Elevate affected limb(s) to reduce swelling.

Chemical burns:

• Remove source of burn (safely remove chemical + clothes in affected area).

• Irrigate the burn with cool (but not iced) running water for **up to 1 hour.**

• Urgent ED review.

Electrical burns:

• SAFELY remove patient from source of burn but if high voltage/unable to switch off power do not approach.

• Urgent ED review.

BURNS ASSESSMENT

Accurate assessment of the following three factors informs how a burn should be managed: [gg]

- SIZE – Total body surface area (TBSA) of the burn
- SITE (or sites) of the body burned
- DEPTH of the burns

Size and Site Assessment

The simplest ways of estimating TBSA are by using the Wallace rule of 9's (Figure 9.1) or the Mersey Burns App.

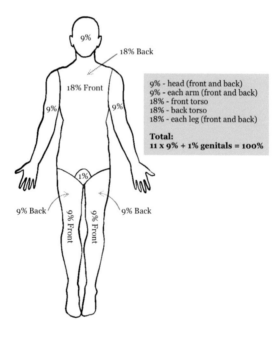

9% - head (front and back)
9% - each arm (front and back)
18% - front torso
18% - back torso
18% - each leg (front and back)

Total:
11 x 9% + 1% genitals = 100%

FIGURE 9.1   Wallace rule of 9s.

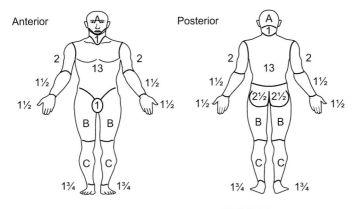

FIGURE 9.2   Lund and Browder chart.

The Mersey Burns App accounts for age and assists in calculating fluid requirements for resus burns. Erythema is not part of the TBSA calculation.

The Lund and Browder chart (Figure 9.2) is also widely used and again accounts for how age affects body proportions so is particularly useful for paediatric burns. The % TBSA is calculated for each separate area taking into account the variation with age in the head, the upper leg and the lower leg (A, B and C).

Depth Assessment

Anatomy of Burn Depths

Superficial	Only outer strata of the epidermis affected (stratum basale preserved). The associated inflammatory response can extend into underlying dermis; however, dermis remains viable.
Mid dermal	Cell death in epidermis and outer layer of dermis with inflammation extending to mid-dermis causing thrombosis of superficial vessels. Skin appendages, fibres, vessels and cells in deeper layer remain viable.
Deep dermal	Cell death to mid dermis and inflammation occurring in reticular dermis with denaturation of the collagen and elastic fibres. All superficial skin appendages destroyed with sparing only of deep hair follicles and vessels.
Full thickness	Burn extends through the full extent of dermis to subcutaneous fat, muscle or even underlying bone. All structures and cells are destroyed throughout skin.

The decision for whether or not surgical intervention is needed relies heavily on the assessment of the depth of a burn (Figure 9.3). Depth is challenging to assess, and also burns evolve over 2–3 days so reassessment is required [hh]. Furthermore, burn wounds are rarely uniform, i.e. some parts superficial some parts deeper.

Depth is assessed by:

1. Appearance of the burn

2. Pain

3. Capillary refill time (CRT)

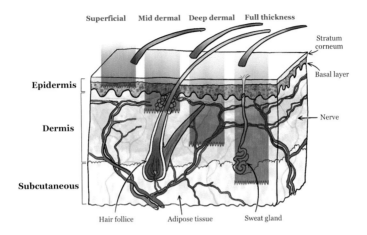

FIGURE 9.3   Burn depths.

A useful method to assess CRT is to take a clean pair of scissors and press the handle on to the burn for 5 seconds then remove quickly. If you can see the blanching outline of the scissor handle, there is a CRT (Figure 9.4). Document if it is normal or slow (slower = more damage).

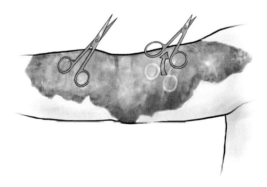

FIGURE 9.4   Assessment of capillary refill time.

Superficial Burns (Epidermal)

Erythematous and warm to touch with brisk capillary refill due to increased dermal vessel blood flow. Typically *painful and do not usually form blisters.* Healing occurs within a few days. Do not scar. Example: Sunburn.

Mid Dermal Burns (Superficial Partial Thickness)

Pale pink in colour with blisters. They are *extremely painful and (when blisters deroofed) blanche with a normal capillary refill.* Healing can take up to 21 days relying on migration of epidermal cells from the wound edges. Despite being unlikely to cause a scar they may temporarily alter skin pigmentation (Figure 9.5).

Deep Dermal Burns (Deep Partial Thickness)

Dark red, often blotchy with no blistering and sluggish (or absent) capillary refill. Typically *are less painful and firmer than more superficial burns.* Healing occurs by contracture resulting in a scar, which can take up to 6 weeks relying on epithelial migration from wound edges and deep hair follicles (Figure 9.6). Scarring likely – takes up to a year to declare fully.

Full Thickness Burns

Skin is dry often leathery, white or charred with no blisters. These wounds do not blanch. Typically not painful due to loss of superficial nerves. Healing (if any) takes more than 4 weeks via contraction and epithelial migration from wound edges. Usually require surgical intervention and

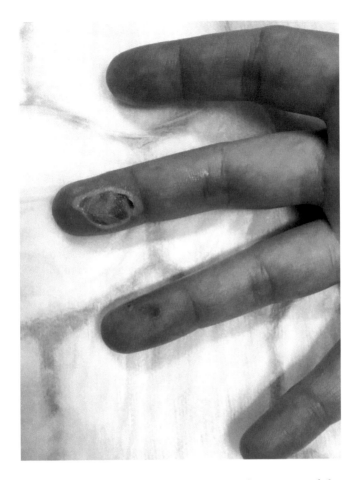

FIGURE 9.5 Superficial partial thickness burn. Deroofed to facilitate assessment then managed with dressings.

always leave a scar (Figures 9.7 and 9.8). If not debrided may lead to functional deficit due to the formation of contractures (tightened scars).

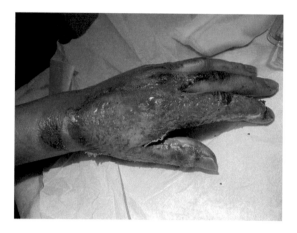

FIGURE 9.6   Mixed mid dermal and deep dermal burn 1-week old. Due to its depth and location over the joints of the index finger the decision was made to excise and skin graft to expedite healing and avoid joint stiffness.

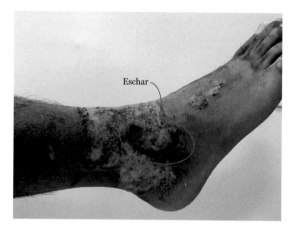

FIGURE 9.7   Deep dermal + full thickness burn 1-day-old. Predominantly deep dermal with an area of eschar. This required excision and split thickness skin grafting.

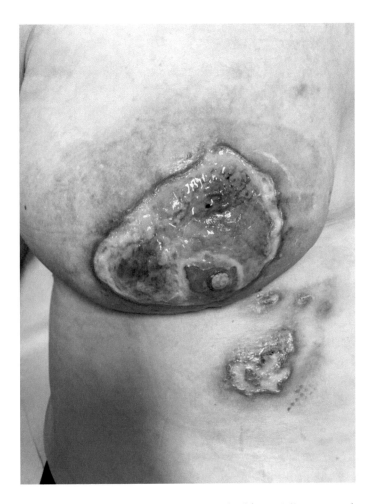

FIGURE 9.8 Full thickness burn 1-week old. Initially managed with flaminol hydro with the aim of non-surgically debriding but when followed up in clinic declared as full thickness so booked for excision and skin graft.

BURNS MANAGEMENT

Minor Burns and Infected Burns

Post first aid and assessment, minor burns can be managed on an outpatient basis. Deroof blisters to allow proper assessment of depth and as they can act as a nidus for infection. Dress the burn appropriately and arrange a review in a burns clinic in 2–3 days to monitor healing. Burns can sometimes become infected – if you are asked to review a potentially infected burn then assess it as you would a cellulitis – looking for erythema around the burn, worsening pain and excessive warmth at the burn site. If there is systemic illness or deranged observations then bloods ± admission for IV antibiotics may be appropriate. If the infection appears minor then wash and dress with an antimicrobial dressing, prescribe oral antibiotics as per local guidelines, give safety net advice and follow up in 2–3 days.

Burns Dressings

The aim of dressing burns is to provide a protective environment to reduce the chance of infection and to minimise protein and fluid loss while the burn heals. A wide variety of burns dressings and topical agents are available, which can make dressing a burn difficult. In addition to this you will find that your senior clinicians have different dressing preferences. That said, remember there are no hard and fast rules and most non-adherent dressings will provide benefit in terms of healing.

There are potentially three components to any burn dressing:

1. Topical agent – May be required.

2. Interface on the surface of the burn – Always required.

3. Overlying dressing – Always required.

Generally speaking, if a burn does not require debridement, moisturising or drying out you should apply a common non-adherent interface (e.g. Adaptic touch or Mepitel), covered by a common dressing (e.g. Softpore/ Biatain/gauze and crepe). If debridement, moisturising or drying out is required you will use something more specialist like a topical agent or an absorptive dressing. The below is a guide to common options as per type of burn.

Superficial Burn

- Do not require dressings – Advise patient to treat with simple non-perfumed moisturisers (e.g. E45, Diprobase) or Vaseline 2–3 times daily. Advise patient to shower daily and pat burn dry.

Mid Dermal Burn (Superficial Partial Thickness – SPT)

- Adaptic touch – Non-adherent silicone interface. Non-absorbent. Lasts up to 5 days.

- Mepitel – Non-adherent silicone interface. Non-absorbent. Lasts up to 5 days. Expensive but good quality.

- Inadine – Antimicrobial mesh interface. Slightly prone to sticking so use a topical agent or other interface such as adaptic touch underneath. Lasts up to 7 days.

- Jelonet – Paraffin gauze. Cheap. Lasts 48 hours after which time dries out and sticks. Best avoided.

- Atrauman – Polyester mesh. Cheap. Tends to stick to burns so best avoided.

- Urgotul silver – Antimicrobial hydrocolloid/silver dressing. Absorbent – Useful in low exudating burns. Lasts up to 7 days.

- Aquacel Ag – Antimicrobial hydrofiber/silver dressing. Absorbent – Useful in exudative burns. Lasts up to 7 days.

- Flaminal forte – Enzymatic alginate gel. Absorbent – Useful on exudative burns and mixed depth burns. Need to apply liberally then overly with dressing such as Aquacel Ag. Lasts up to 3 days.

- Duoderm – Hydrocolloid dressing. Useful on dry non-infected burns requiring moisture ± debridement. Lasts up to 7 days.

- Biatain/Mepilex border. Semi-permeable foam dressings. Absorb + retain moisture.

For example, in a mildly infected but not overly exudative SPT burn you could use an interface like Adaptic touch and overly with an antimicrobial like Inadine or Aquacel Ag interface then apply gauze and crepe on top.

Deep Dermal Burn (Deep Partial Thickness)

- Flaminal forte – Enzymatic alginate gel. Absorbent – Useful on exudative burns and mixed depth burns. Need to apply liberally then overly with dressing such as Aquacel Ag. Lasts up to 3 days.

- Flamazine – Antibiotic (broad spectrum) silver sulfadiazine cream. Breaks down eschar. Apply thinly.

Lasts 24 hours. Caution: Do not use in pregnant and neonates, do not use for >14 days.

- Actilite and activon honey – Antimicrobial topical agent. Breaks down eschar. Lasts up to 3 days.

- Urgotul silver – Antimicrobial hydrocolloid/silver dressing. Absorbent – Useful in low exudating burns. Lasts up to 7 days.

- Aquacel Ag – Antimicrobial hydrofiber/silver dressing. Absorbent – Useful in exudative burns. Lasts up to 7 days.

- Duoderm – Hydrocolloid dressing. Useful on dry non-infected burns requiring moisture ± debridement. Lasts up to 7 days.

- Biatain/Mepilex border. Semi-permeable foam dressings. Absorb + retain moisture.

Full Thickness Burn

Note: In any FT burn, you need to check with a senior if there is indication for surgical management rather than managing with dressings.

- Flaminol hydro – Enzymatic alginate gel. Hydrates and softens eschar rapidly. Can be used over exposed tendons. Lasts up to 2 days.

- Flamazine – Antibiotic (broad spectrum) silver sulfadiazine cream. Breaks down eschar. Apply thinly. Lasts 24 hours. Caution: Do not use in pregnant and neonates, do not use for >14 days.

- Dressings as per mid dermal and deep dermal burns.

Over Granulating (Healing) Burn

- Terra-cortril – Antimicrobial + steroid. Apply thin layer 2–4 times daily.

- Fucibet – Antimicrobial + steroid. Apply thin layer 2–4 times daily.

Specialist Burns Products Unlikely Use in Clinic Setting

- Telfa – Non-adherent plastic – Comes in large sheets, cheap. Normally used in burns theatres to dress large burns post-op.

- Acticoat – Antimicrobial silver mesh. Broad spectrum, very non-adherent. Comes in 3-day and 7-day versions. Expensive.

- Nexobrid – Topical enzymatic debridement agent used by specialists. Acts in 4 hours.

- Biobrane – Biosynthetic dressing: Silicone/nylon mesh + porcine dermal collagen. Used on clean partial thickness burns to encourage skin regeneration.

- Suprathel – Synthetic skin substitute for partial thickness burns. Applied once only and remains on until burn healed. Avoids pain of dressing changes. Commonly used in children.

Resus/Major Burns

Burns >15% TBSA in adults, or greater than 10% in children and the elderly are considered 'resus' burns, i.e. burns that require fluid resuscitation. The systemic sequalae of multiorgan dysfunction are normally associated with burns of >20% TBSA and these burns are considered 'major' burns.

Patients with resus/major burns need to be assessed and managed as per Advanced Trauma and Life Support (ATLS) and Emergency Management of Severe Burns (EMSB) guidelines [ii] [jj]. In a large burn it is easy to miss other injuries, the most important of which is inhalation injury, so keep this in mind when taking the history of the burn and in your assessment of the airway.

Fluid Resuscitation

Fluid resuscitation in burns is as per the Parkland Formula (4 mL × weight in kg × %TBSA burn). For example, for an adult weighing 80 kg with a 16% TBSA burn the calculation would be 4 × 80 × 16 = 5120 mL. This calculation gives the required resuscitation fluid volume required over 24 hours from time of the burn. Half of the total volume should be given in the first 8 hours from the time of burn with the rest given over the next 16 hours. Crystalloids are the fluids of choice (Hartmanns/Plasmalyte) and should ideally be warmed before giving. Most patients will have already been given some fluid by the time you assess them so factor this into your calculation.

This volume does not include maintenance fluids, which will also need to be given if the patient is not drinking. In reality, if a patient is catheterised, the fluid input can be titrated to achieve adequate urine output.

EMSB/ATLS Algorithm

C-SPINE

- Immobilise C-spine until cleared, especially in context of road traffic collision, explosion or electrocution.

- Consider C-spine injuries in patients who are unconscious/intubated/suffering from psychosis/under the influence of substances.

A – AIRWAY

- Facial burn patients should be sat upright to reduce progression of burn associated oedema.

- Ingestion of chemical → immediate anaesthetic assessment ± early intubation.

- Singed facial or nasal hairs, soot in orifices, signs of upper airway compromise such as stridor, respiratory distress, hoarseness, impaired gas exchange, combativeness or decreased level of consciousness (GCS <9) → immediate anaesthetic assessment ± early intubation due to progressively oedematous airway.

B – BREATHING

- 15 litres/min 100% non-rebreathe high flow oxygen and monitor sats.

- Adequate exposure to facilitate assessment of the chest. Circumferential chest burns can restrict ventilation → emergency escharotomy.

- Baseline ABG + carbon monoxide levels (COHb).

- Consider asphyxiant inhalation if there are signs such as lethargy, irritability, severe temporal headache, generalized muscle weakness or CNS depression.

C – CIRCULATION

- Two large bore peripheral IV lines or IO access, preferably through unburned skin + insertion of a urinary catheter to monitor urine output.

- Fluid balance monitoring + resuscitation as per Parkland Formula.

- Baseline bloods (U&E, FBC, LFT, CRP, X-Match, Drug/Tox) + ECG.

- If electrical burn: 12 lead ECG/cardiac monitor is required + CK and myoglogin in blood and urine tests. Aim for high urine output due to increased risk of rhabdomyalosis.

- Routine antibiotic prophylaxis is not recommended.

- Consider nasogastric tube to decompress the stomach/prevent vomiting or aspiration.

D – DISABILITY

- Baseline level of consciousness (e.g. GCS or AVPU).

- Blood glucose.

- In patients with altered level of consciousness or who are irritable consider hypoxia, CO poisoning, shock, associated injury, substance abuse or pre-existing medical conditions as potential reversible causes.

- Analgesia via intravenous opiates in incremental doses until pain is controlled. NSAIDS impact on inflammatory response mediation and can contribute to acute kidney injury so not recommended in resus burns.

E – EXPOSURE/EXTRAS

- Remove dressings, clothing, contact lenses and constricting jewellery near burn.

- Leave any molten or stuck fabrics.

- Irrigate the burn with cool running water (at ≥15°C) for total of 20 minutes. Irrigate the burn only to minimise heat loss. If water supply is limited use cool water compresses – change frequently.

- Segmental approach to cooling extensive burns by cooling one area at any one time to minimise heat loss – remembering to ensuring hypothermia does not occur.

- Chemical burn injuries require prompt and prolonged irrigation. Discuss with senior if neutralising agent such as dipoterine indicated.

- Circumferential burns of limbs and digits may lead to compartment syndrome and may require emergency escharotomies. Elevate affected limb in a Bradford sling and seek senior input re surgical intervention.

- Calculate TBSA.

- Cover irrigated burns with *non-circumferential* strips of cling film or non-adherent dressing.

- For facial burns use a cool water compress (do not apply cling film to face). If burns near eyes → urgent ophthalmology review.

- Check tetanus status and give if not up to date.

Secondary Survey

Do not forget to assess for concomitant injuries by performing a secondary survey.

BURNS EXTRAS

Toxic Shock Syndrome

Toxic shock syndrome (TSS) is a rare, acute, life-threatening illness often associated with burns that is precipitated by bacterial exotoxin release, which can trigger a multisystem inflammatory response progressing to septic shock and multi-organ failure. The most common pathogens are *S. aureus* and Group A *Streptococcus*. Paediatric patients are particularly susceptible to TSS due to their immature immune systems [kk]. TSS generally occurs within 2–4 days of sustaining a burn. The burn itself may have a small TBSA.

The pathophysiology of TSS is a dysregulated host immune response due to the colonisation of a burn wound with toxin-producing strains of bacteria. The most common exotoxin involved is TSST-1 produced by *S. aureus*, which bypasses usual antigen-mediated immune pathways and interacts directly with T-cell receptors stimulating T-cells. The dysregulated response subsequently causes cytokine release which can lead to shock and multi-organ failure [ll]. Definitive testing involves isolation of the exotoxin, which may take many days for the result and so is not useful diagnostically [mm].

Consider diagnosis of TSS in the context of a burn with the following:

- Burn sustained 2–4 days ago
- Pyrexia >39
- Rash (non-specific)
- Diarrhoea ± vomiting
- Irritable/altered behaviour
- Lymphopenia/hyponatremia

Diagnosing TSS is challenging due to the non-specific nature of the presentation. Due to this ambiguity, and the potential severity of TSS, if you have any suspicion of TSS contact your senior immediately to review the patient.

If TSS is suspected, management must be initiated immediately. Involve your consultant + the paediatric team ± critical care (if the child is unstable). Obtain IV access and commence antibiotics for TSS as per trust protocol/micro advice. Fluid resuscitation may be required. In/out balance is strictly required. Patients who are not improving with empirical treatment may be considered for IV fresh frozen plasma (FFP)/IV immunoglobulin (IVIG).

Non-Accidental Injury

All paediatric burns and burns in vulnerable adults should be assessed to rule out non-accidental injury (NAI). A clear history, thorough examination and a knowledge of normal developmental milestones aid assessment of NAI [nn]. If you have any suspicion of NAI either through neglect or deliberate abuse you need to escalate early to an ED consultant and contact the local safeguarding lead who will then manage the case. Ensure this happens *while the patient is in ED* as if they get discharged the assessment cannot be carried out. Fully document your suspicions, reasoning + steps taken. If NAI is suspected in the context of a burn the case should also be discussed with the burns service network as part of the MDT approach.

Suspicion of NAI should be raised by:

- Delay in presentation

- Inconsistent or vague history

- Lack of concern or exaggerated concern about treatment/prognosis

- Burn shape conceivably specific object (iron/cigarette)

- Burns in areas you would not expect to come into contact with heat (soles of feet/buttocks/back/backs of hands)

- Scald with sharply delineated edges (consider immersion injury)

- Depth of burn greater than expected with mechanism of injury

- Presence of old or healing injuries

- Previous social service involvement

Burns Service and Referrals

The national burns service network is made up of *facilities, units and centres* with centres being the highest level of care. Burns service referral (discussion) indications [oo]:

- All burns ≥3% total body surface area (TBSA) in adults and ≥2% in children
- All full thickness burns
- All circumferential burns
- Any burn not healed within 2 weeks
- Any burn injury with signs of infection
- Any cold injury
- Any unwell/febrile child with a burn
- Any burn with a suspicion of non-accidental injury
- Burn injury in pregnant woman
- Burn injuries in patients with pre-existing co-morbidities that could impact management
- Chemical burns
- Electrical burns
- Extremes of age, i.e. neonates, >60 years old
- Inhalation injury (ITU locally if no cutaneous injury)
- Progressive non-burn skin loss condition (necrotising fasciitis, Steven–Johnson syndrome, toxic epidermal necrolysis)

- Special areas – Eyes, face, hands, feet, genitalia, perineum
- Suspicion of toxic shock syndrome

Following discussion with burns specialists, and as a general rule, paediatric burns <5% TBSA or adults with <10% can be managed at a **burns facility**. Burns from 5 to 15% paediatric or >10% to <40% can be managed at a **burns unit**; whilst burn injuries >15% paediatric or adult >40% should be managed at a **burns centre.**

CHAPTER 10

Facial Trauma

Facial trauma comes under the care of Plastics, Maxillo-facial, Ear Nose and Throat (ENT) and ophthalmic surgeons. The way in which the different aspects of facial trauma are divided up depends on what specialties are represented at your unit. In larger hospitals, there is often a designated Maxillofacial team who take all facial trauma, in smaller hospitals it is more common for facial trauma to come to Plastics. Find out the local policy from your colleagues. It is common for ENT to manage septal haematomas, nasal fractures and sometimes pinna haematomas.

When receiving a facial trauma referral, find out BEFORE seeing the patient what other injuries they have. You need to make sure that a serious head injury/C-spine injury/airway compromise has been excluded and that they do not have other significant injuries or illnesses. If they do have other injuries, ensure that relevant referrals have been made and that they are admitted under joint

DOI: 10.1201/9781003163770-10

care with the appropriate specialties. In this way you aim to avoid the 'simple facial laceration' patient who in fact turns out to have multiple medical and surgical problems being admitted under your sole care.

HISTORY

Obtain detailed information about the mechanism of injury as this provides clues about the likelihood of other significant injuries. *Be suspicious for potential involvement of the CNS, the airway and the cervical spine due to their proximity to the face.* A good history gives clues about the facial trauma itself, e.g. level of contamination, likelihood of foreign bodies or likelihood of damage to important structures in the face.

Initial Assessment

If in doubt, assess as per ATLS principles to avoid missing severe injuries. Key points within the ATLS survey are:

Airway

In facial trauma there are several ways in which the airway may be affected:

- Obstruction – Foreign body (teeth, dentures), soft tissue fragments

- Haemorrhage – Oropharyngeal or nasopharyngeal

- Soft tissue swelling

- Facial fractures – Posteriorly displaced maxillary fractures, posterior displacement of the tongue due to mandibular fractures

- Associated laryngeal trauma

Any concern over airway should prompt urgent anaesthetic assessment.

Breathing

- If there is dental trauma obtain a CXR to rule out teeth in the airway.

Circulation and haemorrhage control

- Facial wounds can bleed a lot due to the rich vascularity of the area. To control bleeding sit the patient up (as long as C-spine cleared); apply pressure pack if there is a deep wound. For nasal bleeds attempt to control bleeding by asking the patient to sit slightly forward, blow the nose once to clear clots, then squeeze the soft (alar) portion of the nose for 10 minutes. Don't release the pressure to check prior to 10 minutes elapsing. If this does not control the bleeding the next step is to use a nasal pack (normally available in ED).

- Infiltration of local anaesthetic with adrenaline can aid haemostasis and allow for a more thorough assessment of facial wounds (post initial survey).

Disability

- GCS/AVPU/pupillary response is a key part of CNS assessment. If patient is intoxicated or if for any other reason you cannot assess them seek senior ED input as imaging will likely be required.

FACIAL EXAMINATION

After the primary survey has been completed assess the face in detail.

Inspection

- Global asymmetry/swelling/depressions to face.

- ? Asymmetry of eyes in terms of shape and position (fractures of maxilla/zygoma/orbit can lead to abnormal appearance).

- ? changes in vision (diplopia is suggestive of orbital floor fracture)? loss of any eye movements (again suggestive of orbital fracture). Any concerns – contact Ophthalmology to assess.

- PERLA. Subconjunctival haemorrhage? (skull fracture)

- ? Asymmetry of nose (suggestive of fracture) + look inside nose (septal haematoma = red swelling filling nostril/s).

- Look inside mouth (? Bleeding/obstruction/loose or broken teeth). Check bite for malocclusion.

- If lacerations present assess their depth and likely involvement of key structures:

  - Facial nerve

  - Parotid duct

  - Lacrimal duct

  - External auditory meatus

Palpation

Palpate bilaterally and bimanually to pick up asymmetry.

- Sensation – Decreased sensation over maxilla can indicate infraorbital nerve damage from maxilla or zygoma fracture, numbness of lower lip (inferior alveolar nerve) or chin (mental nerve) suggests mandible fracture. Assess sensation and motor function BEFORE giving local anaesthetic.

- Palpate all bone and soft tissues systematically for tenderness, surface irregularities (foreign bodies), steps (fracture) and swelling (oedema, haematoma).

- Palpate intraorally noting step-offs, lacerations or loose/absent teeth.

Movement

- Test facial nerve motor function (palsy warrants surgical exploration).

FACIAL FRACTURES

If you have any suspicion of a facial fracture (either from the mechanism of injury or your examination findings) obtain imaging. The gold standard for suspected midfacial fractures is CT. For suspected mandibular fractures plain films are adequate. *In any patient who is found to have a facial fracture ensure that a full ATLS primary survey has already been carried out including assessment of the C-spine, airway and CNS as facial fractures are often associated with severe concomitant injuries.* The most common mechanisms causing facial fractures are: Assault, Road traffic collision,

Falls and Sports. The most common facial bones fractured are: Nasal (+ frontal sinus), Mandible, Zygoma and Maxilla. Maxillary fractures are high energy injuries. They are classified as Le Fort 1, 2 and 3 which reflect increasing craniofacial dysjunction. Fractures involving the orbit require urgent ophthalmology review. See below for a summary of common fracture sites and structures affected (Figure 10.1).

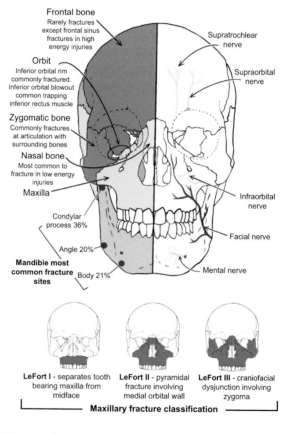

FIGURE 10.1 Common sites of facial fractures.

Most facial fractures need operative intervention because of the functional impairment and deformity that they cause. Always inform the registrar on call about a patient with a facial fracture. All but the most minor facial fractures warrant admission, so if in doubt admit and provisionally prepare the patient for surgery.

FACIAL LACERATIONS

Facial lacerations are best cleaned and closed as quickly as possible to reduce the chance of infection and to minimise deformity. As there is a rich blood supply to the face, skin or tissue flaps with only small pedicles can often survive and the region is relatively resistant to infection. Wounds should be thoroughly irrigated and examined to ensure removal of any foreign bodies or dirt that may tattoo the skin, then conservatively debrided and closed. Layered closure and alignment are important, particularly in aesthetically sensitive areas such as the lip, ear and eyebrow.

Important structures to consider in facial lacerations (Figure 10.2).

- **Lacrimal apparatus**
  - Most commonly associated with medial lower-lid lacerations. Oculoplastic input may be required. If suspected, for senior review + admission for formal repair over a stent (removed after 4–6 weeks).

- **Facial nerve**
  - Essential to test function before the administration of local anaesthetic.

- Suspected facial nerve involvement requires admission for emergency exploration and repair within 72 hours (post 72 hours distal nerve stumps cannot be identified via nerve stimulation).

- Branches medial to the lateral canthus are not routinely repaired and often undergo spontaneous reinnervation; however, discuss these cases with a senior.

- **Parotid duct**

  - Lacerations suspected of involving parotid duct require admission for formal emergency repair (over stent).

- **External auditory meatus**

  - If suspected, for senior review + admission for formal EUA & repair. Circumferential lacerations may require stenting to prevent stenosis.

If you do not suspect damage to any of the above key structures the wound is likely amenable to primary closure under LA in ED. Using local anaesthetic with adrenaline helps control bleeding so makes for easier visualisation and repair (e.g. Lignospan – *2% lidocaine + 1:80,000 adrenaline* or Xylocaine with adrenaline – *1%/2% lidocaine + 1:200,000 adrenaline*). It can be useful to use a regional block for larger lacerations [pp] in addition to local infiltration. Examples of this are supraorbital, infraorbital blocks or mental nerve block.

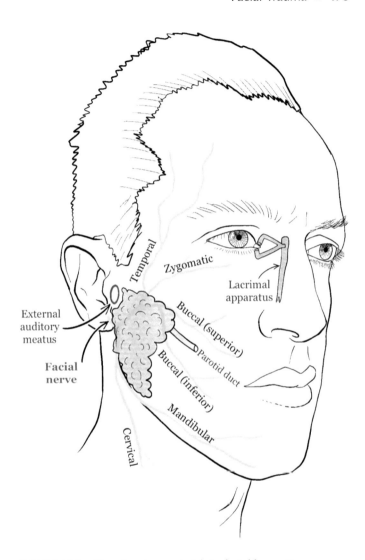

FIGURE 10.2   Key structures at risk in facial lacerations.

Good lighting and loupe magnification make a good quality repair easier.

- Forehead lacerations from falls often penetrate to the periosteum, so it is important to clean these wounds thoroughly and repair the muscle layer as well as the skin.

- In lacerations involving the eyebrow do not shave the eyebrow as it often does not grow back.

- For lacerations of the pinna, repair of the overlying skin and coverage of the cartilage is usually sufficient and suturing through the cartilage is rarely required.

Suture Choice and Suture Removal

- For closure of deeper layers use absorbable sutures, i.e. monocryl or vicryl (4/0 or 5/0 depending on the area).

- For skin use non-absorbable sutures, i.e. prolene or nylon (5/0 or 6/0) to minimise scarring with removal at 5–7 days.

- For younger patients, in which removal of sutures will cause unnecessary trauma, the use of absorbable sutures, i.e. vicryl rapide (6/0 or 7/0) is acceptable.

Paediatric Patients

Children commonly suffer lip lacerations and forehead lacerations due to falls. They vary widely in what they can tolerate – some 6-year-olds happily tolerate LA and some

12-year-olds are unable to. The combination of severity of injury and age of child can make surgical planning tricky so consult a senior if any doubt about the best pathway. LAT gel (lidocaine, adrenaline, tetracycline) can be a very useful topical anaesthetic in children to allow proper assessment ± repair of wounds.

Lip Laceration Repair

The primary goal of lip laceration repair is to align the vermilion border precisely (Figure 10.3).

Repair technique:

1. Manage dental trauma if present + rule out retained foreign bodies.

2. Ensure adequate lighting + ideally use loupe magnification.

3. Mark the vermilion border with a surgical marking pen BEFORE infiltrating anaesthetic, as the volume of anaesthetic will distort the anatomy.

4. Infiltrate local anaesthetic and irrigate wound. If the laceration is large a regional block can also be used (i.e. infraorbital/mental nerve block).

5. Re-approximate orbicularis muscle (if required) using 4/0 absorbable sutures (Monocryl or Vicryl).

6. Place first 2 skin sutures (6/0 nylon/Prolene) either side of marked vermilion border to ensure accurate opposition.

1. Mark vermillion border before injecting LA

2. Repair muscle layer (note swelling due to LA)

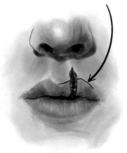
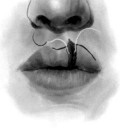

3. Place first skin sutures either side of vermilion border

4. Close externally, then mucosa (if required)

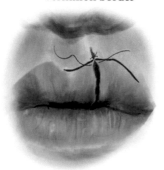

FIGURE 10.3   Repair of lip laceration technique.

7. Close rest of wound with simple interrupted sutures (6/0 nylon/Prolene for skin and 5/0 Vicryl rapide for mucosa). Repair intraoral portion after lip. An assistant is useful for this step.

Post repair:

1. Home with topical chloramphenicol ointment ± oral antibiotics if contaminated ± chlorhexidine mouthwash (if there is a significant intra-oral component).

2. Suture removal in 5 days.

3. Advise use sun protection for at least the next 6 months (>SPF 30) to reduce chance of scarring.

CHAPTER 11

Free Flaps

Free flap reconstruction involves moving tissue from one part of the body to another to reconstruct a defect (Figures 11.1–11.3). The 'donor' tissue is completely disconnected from its blood supply and reconnected to the 'recipient' site blood vessels using microsurgery. There are many possible applications, but are most commonly encountered in the settings of breast, head and neck and lower limb reconstruction.

WHY FREE FLAPS FAIL

Around 5% of free flaps fail due to vascular compromise and resultant ischaemia to the transferred tissue. This happens most commonly within the first 24 hours post-operatively. Close clinical monitoring in the post-operative period is a cornerstone of management of free flaps as prompt recognition of compromise greatly increases the chances of salvaging the flap.

DOI: 10.1201/9781003163770-11 **179**

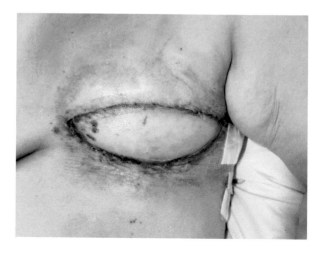

FIGURE 11.1   Healthy flap (left breast deep inferior epigastric perforator flap – DIEP).

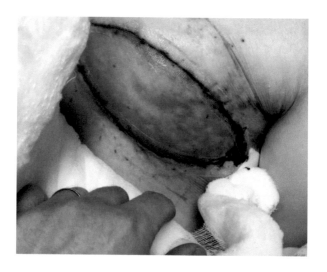

FIGURE 11.2   Flap with venous congestion (left breast DIEP).

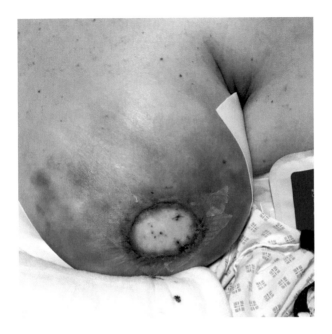

FIGURE 11.3   Flap with compromised arterial inflow (left breast DIEP).

Vascular compromise to the flap can be due to compromise of either the arterial inflow or venous outflow. Arterial failure is usually caused by thrombosis, whereas venous failure may be due to either thrombosis within the anastomosis or extrinsic compression of the vein from, for example, haematoma or vessel kinking.

PRINCIPLES OF FREE FLAP MONITORING

When assessing free flaps, it is essential to have a systematic approach (Figure 11.4), appreciate what a healthy flap looks like (Table 11.1) and be able to recognise signs of arterial or venous compromise early. Most centres have established protocols for monitoring flaps involving nurses performing regular 'flap observations' as well as regular assessments by surgical juniors. You should aim to review free flap patients as soon after the operation as possible (or as soon as you come on call) to help identify any evolving changes during your monitoring period. Juniors should have a low threshold for seeking urgent senior review if they have any concern about a free flap as any signs of compromise should warrant an urgent trip to theatre.

WHAT DOES A HEALTHY FLAP LOOK LIKE?

A healthy flap should be pink in colour, warm to touch, soft, with capillary refill time of 2–3 seconds and audible Doppler signals.

APPROACH TO ASSESSMENT

OPERATION NOTE REVIEW

-Ensure you understand the anatomy of the flap and donor site

⇨ - ? Difficulty performing anastomosis

⇨ - ? Intraoperative blood loss

⇨ - Post-operative Instructions:

- • - Frequency of flap observation
- • - Presence of marker stitch for Doppler signal checking
- • - Preferred nursing position
- • - Intravenous fluid and blood pressure instructions
- • - Anticoagulation instructions
- • - Antibiotic instructions
- • - Patient warming instructions (usually a bair hugger is applied for first 24 hours)

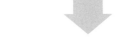

ASSESS HAEMODYNAMIC STATUS

Haemodynamic instability can contribute to flap failure but care should be taken to avoid hypervolaemia as this can cause flap congestion. Discuss with your senior before giving any significant volumes of fluid.

FLAP ASSESSMENT

Review flap observation chart and examine for the following:

- **Colour**

- **Capillary refill time**

- **Temperature**

- **Consistency** (firm/ soft)

- **Doppler signals** - use a handheld doppler to assess arterial blood flow. A marker stitch may have been placed to guide where to apply doppler probe.

+/- Dermal Bleeding - **Only** if there are concerns about the flap - make a scratch to the level of ther dermis to the flap surface using a small needle and see if the flap bleeds readily.

+/- Donor site - the donor site will not need to be reviewed at the same frequency as the flap but should be assessed regularly as complications such as haematoma may also require an urgent trip to theatre.

FIGURE 11.4   Flap assessment flowchart.

MANAGING FLAP COMPROMISE

If you have any concerns about compromise to the free flap alert a senior urgently and prepare the patient for theatre.

TABLE 11.1   Flap Characteristics

	Healthy Flap	Arterial Compromise	Venous Compromise	Irreversible Necrosis
Colour	Pink	Pale, mottled, bluish or white	Cyanotic, bluish or dusky	Fixed purple staining – usually in one part of the flap
Temperature	Warm	Cool	Cool	Cool
Capillary refill time	2–3s	Prolonged	Brisk	Prolonged/absent
Consistency	Soft	Turgor decreased	Tense, swollen	Turgor decreased
Doppler	Good signal	Undetectable	May be detectable in early compromise	Undetectable
+/− Dermal bleeding	Normal flow bright red blood	Minimal bleeding – dark blood or serum	Rapid bleeding – dark blood	Minimal bleeding – dark blood or serum

(Continued)

TABLE 11.1 Flap Characteristics (Continued)

	Healthy Flap	Arterial Compromise	Venous Compromise	Irreversible Necrosis
Immediate management	Continue to monitor as per local flap protocol	• Prepare patient for urgent surgery • Optimise haemodynamically – avoid hypervolaemia • Patient warming • Reposition patient • Loosen bandages +/– on discussion with seniors: • Remove sutures • IV Heparin	• Prepare patient for urgent surgery • Optimise haemodynamically – avoid hypervolaemia • Patient warming • Reposition patient • Loosen bandages +/– on discussion with seniors: • Remove sutures • IV heparin • Leeches	• Prepare patient for urgent surgery • Optimise haemodynamically – avoid hypervolaemia • Patient warming • Reposition patient • Loosen bandages +/– on discussion with seniors: • Remove sutures
Definitive management	–	Immediate Exploration	Immediate Exploration	**Immediate:** immediate exploration **Delayed:** no need for immediate exploration

CHAPTER **12**

Career Development

Plastic surgery is one of the more competitive surgical specialities along with cardiothoracic surgery, neurosurgery, paediatric surgery and maxillofacial surgery. Recruitment takes place annually for ST3 entry and in the 4 years 2017–2020 the average number of UK Plastic Surgery National Training Number jobs (NTN) per year was 36 (range 32–41) and the average competition ratio was 4.12 (range 3.73–4.63) [qq]. The minimum criteria for eligibility to apply is working 6 months within plastic surgery by time of starting ST3 + completion of MRCS exam + completion of core surgery or equivalent. Since the onset of COVID, the recruitment process has altered slightly. Pre-COVID, all candidates who met the eligibility criteria were interviewed and portfolio was marked at time of interview.

From 2021 eligible candidates were asked to upload their portfolios online and these were marked in advance of an interview being offered. The (approximately) 100 candidates whose portfolios scored most highly passed through to the interview stage and selection for NTNs was made from this pool of candidates. The candidates with lower scoring portfolios did not get an interview. The importance of a strong portfolio has thus changed from something desirable to something requisite. At time of writing, it is unknown if this 'portfolio cut-off' will continue in the future or if the system will revert.

Either way it is essential to build a good portfolio to progress to ST3 and this takes time. It is not uncommon for plastics applicants to have started to work on this in medical school. If this is you, great, if not – don't worry, but you do have to start working hard now. Discuss ways to build your portfolio with peers and seniors to learn from others experiences and open doors to potential projects. A lot can be gained by working collaboratively and sharing credit for projects. Think creatively with every project you do, e.g. a good quality audit has the potential to be a poster and also a publication – three birds with one stone. Learn to (politely) say no – avoid complex, poorly defined, long-term projects which require a lot of work for an uncertain return. *Regularly refer back to the portfolio scoring criteria to see if you are working efficiently towards your goals*, and to check you are not missing any low hanging fruit, i.e. things you could easily do to improve your score. Don't worry about things you can't achieve (the PhD) and concentrate on things you can. Collect evidence for things as you go along to avoid missing out on points you deserve. Good luck!

PORTFOLIO SCORING CRITERIA 2021

All fields are rated from A to E. Robust evidence is required to support all ratings. A high rating without evidence of supporting (lower) levels of evidence is unlikely to be accepted.

Included in italics within each table is the overall weighted score that is given to the section. How this is arrived at is not clear to the authors, but the information is useful in so far as to see how important sections are in comparison to each other.

Portfolio scoring criteria and accepted supporting evidence may be subject to change and the authors accept no responsibility for discrepancies between this and any future scoring criteria.

Surgical Experience *(Hands – 8 Marks, Burns – 8 Marks, Skin Cancer – 6 Marks)*					
Hand Trauma	A	B	C	D	E
• Tendon group	No experience	Nail bed repair	Extensor repair (Zones I-VII)	Flexor repair (Zones III-V)	Flexor repair (Zones I-II)
• Fracture group	No experience	MUA hand fracture	K-wire hand fracture	ORIF metacarpal fracture	ORIF phalangeal fracture
• Nerve group	No experience	Suture skin wound	Digital nerve repair	Mixed nerve repair	Nerve graft or nerve transfer
Burns	A	B	C	D	E
• Burns surgery	No experience	Excise and SSG wound <1% TBSA	Excise and SSG wound 1–5%	Excise and SSG wound 6–10%	Excise and SSG wound >10%
• Burns management	No experience	Managed burns <5%	Managed burns 5–10%	Managed burns 10–20%	Managed burns >20%

Skin cancer	A	B	C	D	E
• Skin cancer	No experience	Excise skin malignancy and close directly	Excise skin malignancy and FTSG	Excise skin malignancy and flap closure	Sentinel lymph node biopsy (SLNB)

Supporting evidence: Workplace-based assessments (WBAs) – Ideally consultant level, eLogbook summary signed by consultant, copies of op notes.

Note: (1) No other plastics surgical competencies are judged at ST3 so focus on these three areas of Hands, Burns and Skin Cancer. (2) When you work in burns, do WBAs for burns that you manage! It is natural to focus only on the *surgical* logbook but to score highly you will need evidence of other burns *management*, e.g. clerking, role in resuscitation, wound reviews, decisions on ward rounds, outpatient burns. (3) In 'Burns surgery' you can include SSG to non-burns wounds, e.g. fasciotomy so ensure you log SSGs you perform in other areas of plastics.

Audit *(8 Marks)*				
A	B	C	D	E
No experience	Involved in audit	Completed one audit (including reaudit)	Completed at least one audit every 2 years since graduation. At least 50% should be complete audit cycles including reaudit	Completed at least one audit per year since graduation. At least 50% should be complete audit cycles including reaudit

Supporting evidence: WBAs (ideally consultant level), trust document/ email acknowledging completion of audit/reaudit, poster of audit.

Note: There is no excuse not to get full marks in this section.

Teaching and Training *(8 Marks)*				
A	B	C	D	E
		Collaborator on book chapter	Lead or principle author of book chapter	Editor or author of surgical text book

	eLPRAS author		
Ad hoc medical student or junior doctor teaching	Formal unit or regional teaching presentations	Full time (up to 6 months) formal teaching role or significant formal part-time role	Full time teaching role (greater or equal to 6 months)

Supporting evidence: Book publication details (note: book has to be already published by time of application). eLPRAS link, student feedback, WBAs for teaching presentations, certificate of employment.

Note: There is only 1 overall score for this section, i.e. you could achieve a high score by editing a book OR full-time teaching but if you happen to have done both you don't get double the marks.

Management and Leadership *(4 Marks)*				
A	B	C	D	E
No evidence	Mess president	Departmental rota or management role	Trust/regional and deanery committee or management role	National committees, e.g. Plasta, BMA

Supporting evidence: Letter from dept/trust senior or official body confirming appointment and role.

Higher Qualifications Directly Related to Medicine *(8 Marks)*				
A	B	C	D	E
None	Intercalated BSc awarded or equivalent awarded	Masters with less than 1 year of research awarded	Full-time masters with 1–2 years of research awarded	MD with >2 years of research awarded or PhD awarded

Masters with less than 1 year of research in progress	Full-time masters with 1–2 years of research writing or submitted (lab phase or equivalent complete)	MD with >2 years of full-time research or PhD writing or submitted (lab phase or equivalent complete)	
Full-time masters with 1–2 years of research (lab phase or equivalent in progress)	MD with >2 years full-time research or PhD lab phase or equivalent in progress		
	BDS or equivalent MRCP or equivalent	FDS or equivalent	

Supporting evidence: Letter from supervisor/institution/qualification certificate.

Note: There is only 1 overall score for this section, i.e. 2 degrees at level C would still add up to a C.

Higher Qualifications not Directly Related to Medicine *(4 Marks)*				
A	**B**	**C**	**D**	**E**
None	BSc/BA awarded or equivalent Post Graduate Certificate of Education (PGCert) MA Oxbridge/ Dublin	Masters with less than 1 year of research awarded Masters in Medical Education awarded	Full-time masters with 1–2 years of research awarded	PhD or Doctorate with >2 years full-time research awarded

Masters with less than 1 year of research in progress	Full-time masters with 1–2 years of research writing or submitted	PhD or Doctorate with >2 years full-time research writing or submitted	MBA
Full-time masters with 1–2 years of research (lab phase or equivalent in progress)	PhD or doctorate with >2 years full-time research in lab phase or equivalent		

Supporting evidence: Letter from supervisor/institution/qualification certificate.

Note: There is only 1 overall score for this section, i.e. 2 degrees at level C would still add up to a C.

Academic Prizes and Awards Related to Medicine *(4 Marks)*				
A	B	C	D	E
No experience	Undergraduate prizes and awards including med school finals	Postgraduate prizes/ awards	Regional prizes/ awards	National prizes/ awards

Supporting evidence: Award certificate.

Note: National/international must be the formal conference of a recognised national or international body, e.g. BAPRAS, BSSH, BAHNO and ESPRAS.

PUBLICATIONS AND POSTERS

There are separate tables to fill for the remaining sections. In each you can put multiple entries. Thus, once your work is spread across the sections it can appear thin. Don't be intimidated by this – the majority of candidates will have at the most one or two things in each section. There is no available information on how many entries in each section are required for maximum points.

Publications First Author in a PUBMED Cited Journal *(8 Marks)*				
Title	Authors	Role	Publication Details	Impact Factor

Publications (Not Principal Author) or Principal Author and Not PUBMED Cited *(4 Marks)*				
Title	Authors	Role	Publication Details	Impact Factor

Case Reports/Letters Principal Author *(4 Marks)*				
Title	Authors	Role	Publication Details	Impact Factor

Note: (1) For publications and case reports/letters it is not specified that they have to be related to Plastic Surgery so you can include non-plastics work. (2) There is nowhere to put case reports/letters NOT principle author so only contribute if you can be first author.

International/National Posters Directly Related to Plastic Surgery (**Principal Author**) *(8 Marks between This and Plastics Oral Presentations)*				
Title	Authors	Role	Poster Details	Impact Factor

International/National Oral Presentations Directly Related to Plastic Surgery (Principal Author)				
Title	Title	Title	Presentation Details	Impact Factor

International/National Posters not Related to Plastic Surgery (Principal Author) *(4 Marks between This and Non-plastics oral Presentations)*				
Title	Authors	Role	Poster Details	Impact Factor

International/National Oral Presentations not Related to Plastic Surgery (Principal Author)				
Title	Authors	Role	Presentation Details	Impact Factor

Note: There is nowhere to put presentations/posters NOT principal author so only do projects where you can be first (or joint first).

References

[a] Aldrian S, Nau T, Weninger P, et al. Hand injury in poly-trauma. *Wien Med Wochenschr*. 2005;155:227–232. https://doi.org/10.1007/s10354-005-0173-5

[b] Williams DJ, Walker JD. A nomogram for calculating the maximum dose of local anaesthetic. *Anaesthesia*. 2014 Aug;69(8):847–853.

[c] https://bnf.nice.org.uk/treatment-summary/anaesthesia-local.html

[d] Strazar AR, Leynes PG, Lalonde DH. Minimizing the pain of local anesthesia injection. *Plast Reconstr Surg*. 2013 Sep;132(3):675–684.

[e] Thomson CJ, Lalonde DH, Denkler KA, Feicht AJ. A critical look at the evidence for and against elective epinephrine use in the finger. *Plast Reconstr Surg*. 2007 Jan;119(1):260–266

[f] Janis J (Ed). Essentials of plastic surgery, 2nd edition. *QMP/CRC*. 2014:964–965.

[g] Francel T, Marshall K, Savage R. Hand infections in the diabetic renal transplant patient. *Ann Plast Surg*. 1990;24:304–309.

[h] Gaines RJ, DeMaio M, Peters D, Hasty J, Blanks J. Management of contaminated open fractures: A comparison of two types of irrigation in a porcine model. *J Trauma Acute Care Surg*. 2012;72(3):733–736. doi: 10.1097/TA.0b013e318239caaf.

[i] Kennedy CD, Lauder AS, Pribaz JR, Kennedy SA. Differentiation between pyogenic flexor tenosynovitis and other finger infections. *Hand (N Y)*. 2017;12(6):585–590. doi: 10.1177/1558944717692089.

[j] Shoji K, Cavanaugh Z, Rodner CM. Acute fight bite. *J Hand Surg Am*. 2013;38(8):1612–1614. doi: 10.1016/j.jhsa.2013.03.002.

[k] Janis J (Ed). Essentials of plastic surgery, 2nd edition. *QMP/CRC*. 2014:973.

[l] Koshy JC, Bell B. Hand infections. *J Hand Surg Am*. 2019;44(1):46–54. doi: 10.1016/j.jhsa.2018.05.027.

[m] NINJA clinical trial in progress at time of press

[n] Landin ML, Borrelli MR, Sinha V, Agha R, Greig, AVH. *Composite grafts for fingertip amputations: A systematic review*. *IJS: Short Reports*. 2021 Jan/Mar;6(1):e17. doi: 10.1097/SR9.0000000000000017.

[o] British Society for Surgery of the Hand Guidelines. https://www.bssh.ac.uk/bssh_standards_of_care_in_hand_trauma_.aspx

[p] Janis J (Ed). Essentials of plastic surgery, 2nd edition. *QMP/CRC*. 2014:785–800.

[q] Abzug J, Dua K, Sesko B A, Cornwall R, O Wyrick T. Pediatric phalynx fractures. *J Am Acad Orthop Surg*. 2016 Nov;24(11):e174–e183.

[r] Welman T, Popova D, Vamadeva SV, Pahal GS. Management of amputated digits. *Br J Hosp Med (Lond)*. 2020 Nov 2;81(11):1–8.

[s] Gault DT. Extravasation injuries. *Br J Plast Surg*. 1993;46(2):91–96. doi: 10.1016/0007-1226(93)90137-Z.

[t] Maly C, Fan KL, Rogers GF, et al. A primer on the acute management of intravenous extravasation injuries for the plastic surgeon. *Plast Reconstr Surg Glob Open*. 2018;6(4):e1743. doi: 10.1097/GOX.0000000000001743.

[u] Misiakos EP, Bagias G, Patapis P, Sotiropoulos D, Kanavidis P, Machairas A. Current concepts in the management of necrotizing fasciitis. *Front Surg*. 2014;1:36.

[v] Fernando SM, Tran A, Cheng W, et al. Necrotizing soft tissue infection: Diagnostic accuracy of physical examination, imaging, and LRINEC score: A systematic review and meta-analysis. *Ann Surg.* 2019;269(1):58–65.

[w] Parenti GC, Marri C, Calandra G, Morisi C, Zabberoni W. Necrotizing fasciitis of soft tissues: Role of diagnostic imaging and review of the literature. *Radiol Med.* 2000;99(5):334–339.

[x] Singh P, Khatib M, Elfaki A, Hachach-Haram N, Singh E, Wallace D. The management of pretibial lacerations. *Ann R Coll Surg Engl.* 2017;99(8):637–640.

[y] Lo S, Hallam MJ, Smith S, Cubison T. The tertiary management of pretibial lacerations. *J Plast Reconstr Aesthet Surg.* 2012;65(9):1143–1150.

[z] https://www.boa.ac.uk/standards-guidance/boasts.html. See PDF on Open Fractures (2017).

[aa] Kehoe A, Smith JE, Edwards A, Yates D, Lecky F. The changing face of major trauma in the UK. *Emerg Med J.* 2015;32:911–915.

[bb] von Keudell AG, Weaver MJ, Appleton PT, Bae DS, Dyer GSM, Heng M, Jupiter JB, Vrahas MS. Diagnosis and treatment of acute extremity compartment syndrome. *Lancet.* 2015 Sep 26;386(10000):1299–1310.

[cc] National Network for Burn Care. *National Burn Care Referral Guidance*, 2012. https://www.britishburnassociation.org/national-burn-care-referral-guidance/

[dd] Australia and New Zealand Burn Association. Burn wound assessment. In: *Emergency Management of Severe Burns Course Manual*, 10th edition. Albany Creek: Australia and New Zealand Burn Association Ltd, 2006:42–47.

[ee] Hettiaratchy S, Papini R. Initial management of a major burn: II – Assessment and resuscitation. *BMJ.* 2004;329:101–103.

[ff] American College of Surgeons. *Advanced Trauma Life Support: ATLS Student Course Manual*, 9th edition. American College of Surgeons: Chicago, 2012.

[gg] Battaloglu E, et al. Faculty of Pre-Hospital Care and British Burn Association Expert Consensus Meeting: Management of Burns in Pre-Hospital Trauma Care. [Online], 2020. https://fphc.rcsed.ac.uk/media/2957/2020-09-20-burns-consensus.pdf

[hh] Young AE, Thornton KL. Toxic shock syndrome in burns: Diagnosis and management. *Arch Dis Child Educ Pract.* 2007;92:97–100. doi: 10.1136/adc.2006.101030.

[ii] Chuang YY, Huang YC, Lin TY. Toxic shock syndrome in children: Epidemiology, pathogenesis, and management. *Pediatr Drugs.* 2005;7(1):11.

[jj] Childs C, Edwards JV, Dawson M, Davenport PJ. Toxic shock syndrome toxin-1 (TSST-1) antibody levels in burned children. *Burns.* 1999;25:473–476.

[kk] Chester DL, Jose RM, Aldlyami E, King H, Moiemen NS. Non-accidental burns in children – Are we neglecting neglect? *Burns.* 2006;32:222–228.

[ll] NHS Specialised Commissioning. National Burn Care Referral Guidance, 2012. https://www.britishburnasso-ciation.org/national-burn-care-referral-guidance/

[mm] Zide BM, Swift R. How to block and tackle the face. *Plast Reconstr Surg.* 1998;101(3):840–851.

[nn] https://specialtytraining.hee.nhs.uk/Competition-Ratios

Index